Strong Like A Mother

A postpartum survival guide for working out, navigating injury, and giving yourself grace when your baby arrives.

WRITTEN BY
DR. LAUREN HEINEN, DPT

DEDICATION

To making the world a better place for the moms that hold us dear

ACKNOWLEDGEMENTS

I would like to express my gratitude for all of the help received to make this very special book a reality.

To Tiffany Bailey for the excellent editing, Tashbii and Pelvic Guru, LLC for the lovely figure illustration and to Scott Parrish for the layout work and for designing a beautiful cover that speaks to my heart.

To my family for giving me the support to follow this dream and dedicate myself to the writing process.

And to the mothers in my life who inspire me to be better and to be the strongest version of myself.

Thank you to everyone!

TABLE OF CONTENTS

Introduction

Hi gang! My name is Lauren Heinen. I am a Doctor of Physical Therapy and a mama who specializes in women's health and orthopedics. I have been very passionate about maternal wellness and making sure our mamas-to-be and current mamas are happy, healthy people inside and out. As a fellow mom, I have experienced a wide range of these emotions and physical conditions myself and treat many in my clinic for the same concerns day in and day out. It is such a privilege to get the opportunity every day to speak to and help these beautiful women who sacrifice so much to bring tiny humans into the world.

I am using this book as an opportunity to debunk some of the lesser-known facts and happenings surrounding the postpartum period. In my experience, both professional and personal, I have encountered a lot of "nice to know" things and have had so very many conversations with patients and friends about things we "wish we knew more about" before having babies.

There are so many books for when you are pregnant and what to expect when your body is going completely nuts while growing the next number on the census, but there is a gap in the market when it comes to what to do with yourself after the baby arrives.

You see your OB at two weeks postpartum for a checkup and then again at 6 to 8 weeks postpartum, then you get the "all clear."

All clear for what? Professional rugby? Or just getting back to more of your daily activities? What if we want to move before the 6-week mark?

How do we know where to draw the line? What if you were an athlete before birth? When is it safe to go back to that?

I will lean into the treatment of physical conditions in the postpartum period, as that is my clinical area of expertise, as well as addressing safety regarding returning to sports and exercise following all types of births. I am going to touch on other things, such as physiological conditions (like lochia and swelling of the legs), maternal mental health (mostly concerning knowing that you're not alone in how you're feeling), postpartum nutrition, and, of course, parenting like a boss! Since these are not in my scope as a medical professional, I will do my best to provide a current snapshot of what research tells us and provide advice and resources to refer anyone wanting more information from the appropriate professional.

Treating this population of patients is so special to me, and I feel so passionate about educating people and caring for them during this vulnerable time in their lives. I strive to be someone who can help guide them and give them answers. It makes my heart so happy to be able to interact and connect with women who are navigating this new and awesome time in their families' lives. I feel so lucky to be a person with whom a new mother can share something as significant as her birth story, her joys, and her challenges. Before I had kids, I loved working with this population and felt compassionate toward new moms. When I had kids myself and was given the insight and empathy into what it really feels like, I knew I had to step up my game and really show up for the postpartum community.

Birth is an incredibly significant experience, and I really wanted to create something to help new parents navigate it a little better, laugh together, and, most importantly, show women that they are not alone. We are definitely stronger together.

Thanks for joining me on this journey. You got this, mama—there is nothing quite like being strong like a mother!

CHAPTER ONE:

You survived an entire human (or humans!) exiting your body. Now what?

Congratulations on your bundle of joy! Here is a 9-pound bowling ball with arms and legs that you have to expertly keep alive while you recover from one of the wildest physical events your body will ever accomplish in the span of your lifetime. And FYI, this bundle of joy does not sleep, you will be using your body to feed it every two hours, and it is imperative to make sure you're getting plenty of rest, water, and good nutrition.

It's hard to look back and remember what life was like before this incredibly significant moment and to know who and how to be as a new mom. An entire identity shift (and, in my case, a crisis) begins the moment you deposit your tiny human into the world.

There's no instruction manual, and the last time I checked,
What to Expect After What You've Been Expecting Has
Arrived does not exist to tell you all of the do's and don'ts of
new motherhood. It is a huge change.

In fact, research shows that your baby's cells remain in your body postpartum through microchimerism, a super cool concept where fetal cells pass through the mom's blood and are deposited in organs. So, you have actually changed on a cellular level just by creating this human (Gammill et al.).

Multiple studies have been done on the brains of postpartum females showing a change in the size of neurons in different parts of the brain, and it is said that memory and learning ability improve, even though "mom brain" will fight this concept rather intensely, causing you to lose your train of thought mid-sentence (Rijnink et al.).

You may be thinking, "I know a lot of moms," and even have friends or family members that have become moms. But then, all of a sudden, they hand you your own human and kick you out into the cold, harsh world, and it's time to panic a little.

So, where do we even begin to sort things out? What does it even mean to be postpartum, and how do we get back to a place where we feel at home in our new identity while still feeling like ourselves?

The postpartum period is an absolutely amazing time spent with your baby—finally on the outside!—that you could not imagine loving more, but if we're being honest, it can be very overwhelming. The acute postpartum period includes the first 24 hours following birth, the subacute phase includes the first 6 to 8 weeks following birth, and the late phase includes the period of 6 to 8 months following birth. A lot of healing and changes occur physically and mentally during these different phases. In fact, this whole journey of physical and mental changes started well before the moment you delivered your baby.

Let's break down the last 40 or so weeks of your life, culminating in the magical moment we call birth.

First, you conceive a child. Then, over the next 38 weeks or so, your body rapidly changes to literally grow another walking, talking, loving little person. The uterus grows from the size of an orange to the size of a literal watermelon, your blood volume increases by about 35%, body weight increases by an average of 30-40 pounds, weird hair grows in places you never knew were possible, your abdominal and pelvic floor muscles will stretch and experience incredible amounts of stress, and new waves of hormones are rapidly pumping through your body constantly. It's the wild west of body changes all in about ten months' time. And that's just growing the kid.

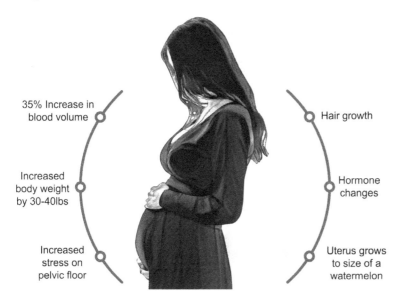

35% Increase in blood volume

Hair growth

Increased body weight by 30-40lbs

Hormone changes

Increased stress on pelvic floor

Uterus grows to size of a watermelon

FAST FORWARD TO BIRTH.

For many, the birthing experience is beautiful and significant, but it is a marvel of a physical feat. Some women labor and have contractions for hours on end before pushing a baby out of an opening that previously was NOT the size of a baby. Or perhaps, a c-section occurred—or as my husband likes to call it, a "country club birth" (he's a hilarious man).

> *Either way, something extremely physically significant happened, and you are now left with the aftermath of a body that previously contained a tiny human living on the inside, who now lives on the outside.*

It's wild. What's even crazier is that our bodies begin to rapidly start changing back to their previous state.

TYPES OF BIRTHS

Not every birth is the same, but all are equally valid. Here are the various ways you might bring your new little bundle of joy into the world.

VAGINAL BIRTH

A vaginal birth occurs when a mother goes into labor and delivers her baby through the birth canal. A vaginal birth can look different from family to family, ranging from no epidural to the use of an epidural. Whatever way you choose to bring your child into the world is valid. Birth is HARD, and there is no "easy way out."

In a regular vaginal birth, the pelvic floor will experience a great deal of stress and often can become injured in birth via a perennial tear. Some births may include an episiotomy, which is a small surgical incision to the perineum to help assist the baby in exiting the vaginal canal.

> *No matter what, the pelvic floor post-birth will need some time to recover.*

This muscle group was stretched and supported the weight of a growing uterus for many months. (Imagine setting a bowling ball in a hammock for an extended period of time!) Additionally, the role of the hormone relaxin comes into play to widen and separate the bones of the pelvis as needed to allow the baby to exit the birth canal. It is not uncommon for women to experience lumbopelvic pain, pelvic floor dysfunction (including pain with sexual intercourse, also referred to as dyspareunia), incontinence, or prolapse following vaginal birth.

CESAREAN SECTION

In a cesarean section birth, an incision is made in the lower abdominal area, and it's necessary to get through and move around about eight different layers of tissues: skin, adipose (fat tissue), the external obliques, the internal obliques, the rectus abdominis, the transverse abdominis, the broad ligament, and lastly, the final incision to the uterus itself. Typically, in a planned c-section, the anesthesiologist will place a spinal block to numb the lower body while the mother stays awake for the birth. Mom will have to stay in bed with a catheter for about 24 hours post-delivery as sensation and motor function return to the lower body. Following this period, it is very important for mom to start mobilizing—such as sitting up at the edge of the bed and walking as tolerated with assistance—all while being careful of protecting the incision of her surgical site. Since the abdomen was cut for surgery, some pain with functional movement will occur, as the core is responsible for performing and helping with a lot of these things and will be impaired at this time. This is going to get better, I promise—and I would know as a two-time C-section veteran myself. Following a c-section, it is not uncommon for a woman to experience issues like abdominal pain, scar tissue problems around the incision, abdominal dyskinesia, and lumbopelvic pain, just to name a few.

We are going to discuss post-birth conditions more in Chapter 3 and how to manage them efficiently.

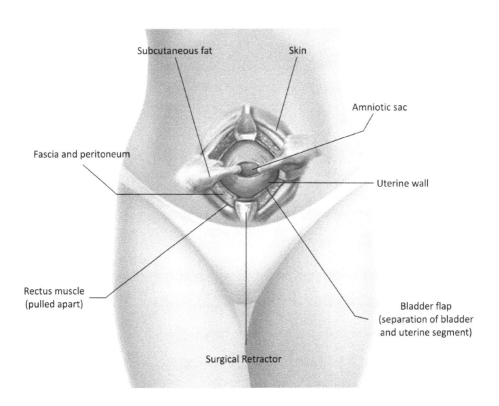

CHANGES IN THE POSTPARTUM PHASE

The postpartum phase, or "puerperium," lasts about six weeks to 6 to 8 months as our organ systems return to their recovered pre-pregnancy states. The uterus takes about six weeks to return to normal size. During that time period, bleeding called lochia (or "not your period") will occur, which is a real bummer if you have a summer baby like my second child was because swimming is off the table until that bleeding stops. This bleeding is somewhat like menstruation, but it instead reflects the changes of the uterus, cervix, and vagina back to their normal status. Also, note that many of your other systems will be making their way back to "normal" as well, such as your renal system (still peeing like crazy? I know, it's not fair) and cardiovascular system as your blood volume, blood pressure, and heart rate all normalize.

BREASTFEEDING

Mammogenesis, or the preparation of the body to breastfeed, begins during pregnancy and really gets kicked up a notch postpartum when it's finally time to feed the baby. All science aside for a second,

no one told me that breastfeeding was hard. Like really hard.

Before I had my first baby, I thought, "Hey, mothers have nursed their newborns since the beginning of time. This is going to be so natural and easy; let's skip the class on it. I need a nap instead."

HELLO, HUMBLING EXPERIENCE.

For some, it may come easy. For others, not so much. For some, it's just not an option for medical or psychological reasons. Whatever you choose, it's the right choice for you and your baby. Don't let anyone bully you into thinking you're not doing something right because you choose to feed your baby differently from someone else. The best way to feed your baby is whatever makes them happy, healthy, and fed. There's a lot of intensity surrounding feeding a baby, and this can come with a lot of pressure from others trying to push you into doing what they think is best. However, they are not you or your partner and don't get to boss you around.

MENTAL HEALTH

Mentally, the period after birth can be overwhelming for a lot of different reasons, with the obvious factor being that you are responsible for keeping a tiny, sweet pea little babykins alive. Also, there is a distinct shift in hormones in a short period of time in the acute postpartum phase that can lead to postpartum depression or its little cousin, the baby blues. The difference between the two is really based on the length of time the symptoms last. Baby blues are similar symptoms of feeling overwhelmed, depressed, or incapable, but the feelings end before the two-week postpartum mark when the mother begins to feel more like herself. Postpartum depression will last longer and can be managed with medication and talk therapy.

I am so passionate about the postpartum mental state of mothers and advocating for making people feel heard and like they are not alone. I think that the medical community is doing a better job of checking in with moms postpartum, and some pediatricians are even including a postpartum depression screen at the first few newborn visits.

We have to break the stigma surrounding maternal mental health and take care of our mamas.

NUTRITION

It can be hard to know what to eat or how much to move following birth. Appetites can increase or decrease, movement can hurt, or maybe you're feeling exhausted from not sleeping and feel like you will never sleep again (it gets better, trust me). If someone was an athlete before having a baby, when would it be safe for them to get back to working out? These questions are important and need to have more criteria and guidelines so that the postpartum community, as well as the wellness community, can safely help with the return to movement.

It is perfectly okay to have mixed feelings about your body after the birth of your baby.

It is perfectly okay to feel at home in your new body. It's okay to feel acceptance for your new body, and it's okay to grieve for the way your body felt and looked before having a baby. It is okay to be overwhelmed, and it's okay to be proud of yourself that you have that babykin's schedule down! That is all valid! You may have all of these feelings in a single day. A lot of changes just happened. The important thing to remember is that you have made it this far and have brought a beautiful new life into the world. It's okay that things feel different because they ARE different and in wonderful ways. Let's normalize being okay with who and where we are with the process. Some days, you may just need to let yourself feel bummed out about not being able to run a 5K as fast as you could before having your baby, and some days, you may look in the mirror and embrace your stretch marks as badass tiger stripes that signify the toughest thing you've endured. Each day might be different, and instead of rushing yourself to get to a place reminiscent of where you were prior to having your baby, you can land on savoring and enjoying each day as it comes, knowing that you can make it through tough things and on to tomorrow.

In the following chapters, I am going to share a lot of personal anecdotes and anecdotes of patients and friends in the hope that you can relate and feel less alone in the experience of motherhood—or if you're reading as a support person to a mother, provide some insight of the things that can go on for you to better support your loved one. I will also share standards of care and resources in the medical, mental health, and wellness fields in order to help guide and direct anyone who may need more information or help.

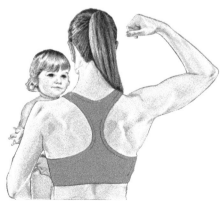

CHAPTER TWO:

"No one told me that was going to happen!" and other various logistics for the days following birth

My first daughter was born via emergency c-section. Everyone is happy and healthy now, but what a rough start for such a tiny human and, in the spirit of being vulnerable, me! My birth plan included doing an unmedicated hospital delivery. Knowing what I know now, I have a lot of trouble recounting this information about that birth story with a straight face. It was disastrous. It resulted in me standing in the corner of my delivery room bathroom like a feral animal clutching to the grab bars as my husband and labor and delivery nurse tried to coax me out and back into the bed. That day was an excellent lesson in doing things my daughter's way, and that remains consistent now as she reigns over our home in her "threenager" dictatorship.

That day was the first instance to start teaching me a lot about letting go of my parental expectations and plans for a lot of things.

Following the c-section, I had a lot of different feelings that were quite intense. At first, I had assumed that it was just a result of being all keyed up from the adrenaline and medication, but a few days passed, and I still felt unlike myself mentally. I was crying a lot and had little control over my emotions. I felt very inadequate and was easily overwhelmed by stimuli and sensory input. Each day that this persisted, I began to panic more. It was like being stuck in the brain of someone else. I knew who I wanted to be and how I wanted to act, but my brain wouldn't allow it. I was worried that I would never be the same again.

My OB/GYN, a saint amongst women, gave me the best pep talk in the hospital when I expressed my concerns to her. She said it was going to take time, that it happens to a lot of moms (herself included), and that whatever happened, we would handle it together.

I had "the baby blues."

Baby blues is a very similar condition to postpartum depression and is classified by lasting less than a two-week period following giving birth.

Anything longer than this is classified as postpartum depression. Day nine postpartum, I was sobbing at the kitchen sink, baby bottles in hand, telling my husband that I was afraid some weird bacteria would get in them and make the baby sick. I woke up on the tenth day, and it was as if someone snapped their fingers, and I was back. Something like this was not even on my radar for occurring after the baby was born. I still look back to that period in awe that I did not see it coming.

I share this in the hopes that anyone else who has gone through it will know that if this does happen, it's okay. Everything is going to get better, and I hope you have a wonderful support system like the one I was so fortunate to have. If you don't, reach out to local services that are available to new moms! So many of the postpartum patients I treat have similar stories. I am not a mental health professional, but I still have an hour-long session with each patient, and I hope to give them a safe, pressure-free environment to express themselves and talk about the things that may be weighing on their minds and lead them to the appropriate resources if needed.

If you're expecting, these are some things you can discuss with your OB/GYN to have a contingency plan in place in the event that it happens. Medically, we know that mothers with a history of depression or anxiety are at a higher risk for developing postpartum depression, postpartum anxiety, or the baby blues after giving birth. These aren't things to actively worry about, but they are things to be aware of and to plan for if needed.

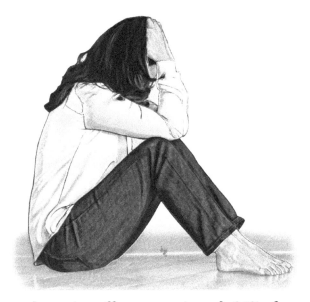

Postpartum depression affects approximately 20% of new mothers.

That's one out of five women who give birth. You are not alone in facing this. Postpartum depression can be managed and lessened with some serious self-care: good sleep, a good diet, good hydration, exercise, and getting out of the house. A lot of these things are tough to come by in the newborn period. Trust me—that is not lost on me. Later, I will talk about the "newborn vortex," where time and space don't exist, and showers are a hard 'maybe.' But the more you fill your cup, the more you will have to work with.

Small steps to taking care of yourself are a great place to start. Open the shades, chug some water while you're pumping, take some deep breaths in the shower, or go for a walk. Anything you can do to take some time to take good care of yourself counts. Furthermore, PPD can be treated with talk therapy, such as cognitive behavior therapy and interpersonal therapy, or it can also be treated pharmacologically with medications such as anti-depressants and anti-anxiety medications. We have to work together to break the stigma surrounding mental health, specifically maternal mental health. No one is judging you. If you need help, reach out to your support system, talk to a friend that makes you feel good, hug someone you love, and most importantly, don't hesitate to call your doctor. We have all been there, and there is no shame in recognizing that you need help to get back to being in a better place.

Screening for postpartum depression is very important as well as giving new moms the opportunity to talk about how they are really feeling. Having a newborn can be overwhelming, and depression is a serious, clinical issue. A good resource to check out is the Edinburgh Postnatal Depression Scale. It's a 10-question screen that just helps to check in with how a new mom is feeling. This is a nice barometer to complete every few weeks or if you're feeling significantly more blue all of a sudden ("Screening"). Don't be ashamed if postpartum depression is a stop on your postpartum journey. With the right treatment and resources, this can be managed.

> *You deserve to be your best you, not only for your little humans that need you but also for you! You're worth it to feel good in your own mind and body.*

I still recall the birth of my first daughter and have big feelings about it. It was a really traumatic day. My emotions ranged from being terrified, being grateful we all made it safely, feeling guilt for not giving her a better experience with coming into the world, and also heaps of anxiety afterward. It helped (and still helps) to talk to others about the experience, and there was a great strength that came with sharing my experience with others. Talk it out with friends. Use your village, not just for baby but for you as well!

PHYSIOLOGICAL RECOVERY

I want to start by declaring that I strongly encourage being body positive following birth. However, it was a slight surprise when I took a first glance in the mirror whilst still in the hospital to see that I still looked super pregnant—big belly, sausage ankles, puffy feet, and pretty much a "Violet from Willy Wonka" situation going on without the blueberry hue. As an emotional human, I was upset. I spent such a long time being pregnant that, by the end, I could not wait to have my body back to not sharing it with someone else. Here is another piece of historical Lauren information that, in retrospect, is laughable because infants are, in fact, akin to tiny barnacles.

To start recovering and looking and feeling more like "myself," I got home from the hospital and could not wait to weigh myself, as baby plus placenta and everything else that just came out weighs approximately 15 pounds. That first glimpse at the scale, and I was only three pounds less than my last logged pregnancy weight. I had retained water post-c-section like it was my job. When I tell you there was foot swelling, it wasn't like anything I had experienced during my pregnancy—they were voluminous. It took about a week with my first and closer to two weeks with my second, but eventually, all of the swelling decreased, and I gladly welcomed back the sight of my ankle bones.

Following the great swelling flush, my body resembled an empty potato sack. It's worth repeating again that I encourage being body positive, but just like anything else, it takes work to get there mentally. Find something you like about yourself (hey there, cute ankle bones!) and build from there. It's going to take some time for your body to recover musculoskeletally, endocrinologically, cardiovascularly, and all of the other systems, too.

> *If a friend broke their ankle, you wouldn't expect them to get up and dance a fancy jig the day after, so give yourself a minute, too.*

We transition into and out of pregnancy not all at once but gradually and at our own pace. It's easy to see someone else's progress and feel the need to compare.

Some of the very best postpartum tips and tricks have been given to me by my prenatal and postpartum patients. For my friends who have had a vaginal delivery, "padcicles" (gigantic frozen maxi pads) will be a great thing to invest in. You can buy some at the store or make your own! Following vaginal birth, there will be bruising, swelling, and (potentially) different degrees of tearing to the perineum. It's a warzone down there. Logistically, this will cause some discomfort with sitting and using the restroom. In fact, most hospitals won't let you leave following a vaginal delivery until you've successfully completed a bowel movement. Icing the area will help reduce inflammation and pain. I would also recommend becoming familiar with how to use a peri bottle. The peri bottle, or "poor man's bidet," will help to gently keep this area clean for good hygiene and proper wound management.

My c-section sisters! For your first night home in your own bed, you won't have bed rails to help you get in and out of bed. All four layers of the abdominals were moved around in the birthing procedure, and you will have an incision to work around and take care of. We use our core for all of our functional movement—something you will become acutely aware of following this experience. I recommend getting a pillow wedge to elevate your head to make it easier to sit up and to learn how to perform "the log roll." This is going to take as much stress as possible off of your core with getting up and down. Accept a helping hand from your partner. Every two to three hours, you will be getting up to feed the baby, and you're going to want to optimize strategies for moving around as pain-free and efficiently as possible.

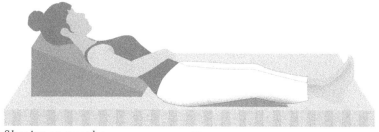

Sleeping on a wedge

I think one of the main things I hear or get questions about are people who are concerned about hurting the incision area by moving around too much. This is, again, something to be aware of, but not something you should let live rent-free in your brain. Unless your doctor specifically orders bed rest, you're going to want to be up and moving as much as you can tolerate in a safe and reasonable manner to prevent blood clots, pneumonia, and atelectasis. I am going to go over exercising later in Chapter 4, but you're going to want to try and walk as much as you can. This sometimes means just the 20 feet to the bathroom and back a few times a day. Body moving, blood flowing. You can increase that distance in small intervals and listen to your body when it tells you to "stop" when things start to hurt. Another criteria to keep in mind is the amount of bleeding or "lochia" that occurs. If there is a sharp increase in bleeding and you are bleeding through a max absorbancy pad in less than two hours, call your doctor right away.

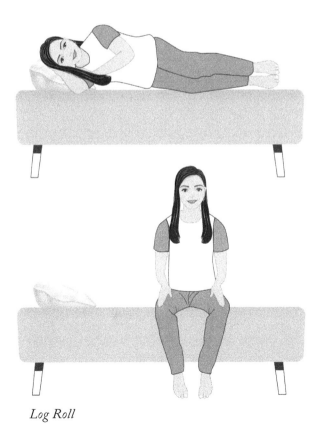

Log Roll

THE NEWBORN VORTEX

I like to refer to the two weeks following the birth of both of our babies as "The Newborn Vortex."

You don't know what time or day it is, can't pin down the time and place of your last shower or meal, and have turned into a "mom vampire" who no longer really sleeps.

The sole purpose of existing is to keep your children alive. It is really crazy and hectic, and it can feel very isolating at times, especially at night. I can recall feeling panicked when the sun would go down in anticipation of knowing I was not going to sleep that night. When I had my second baby, my friend Kirsten, who had recently given birth, told me to text her in the middle of the night at any time because she would be up, too. That small gesture made me feel so much less alone.

My mom pro tip for those with babies 8-12 weeks and under: set an iPad and ear pods next to your feeding station and watch some hilarious sitcoms or other shows on Netflix when you're rocking the baby to sleep. My first baby was born right before Christmas, so you can take it to the bank that I watched Hallmark holiday movies obsessively because I love love and Christmas.

A big question from a lot of people outside of "The Newborn Vortex" is whether or not to visit the newly grown family. I can remember every sweet gesture of food and people stopping by to say hi, making us feel loved, and giving us well wishes. Yes, I was tired and probably very dirty (there is a significant lack of showers in the vortex), but I was going to be up all of the time anyway. I may as well have enjoyed the company of a good friend. I never felt like I needed to entertain them; it just felt good to be and to enjoy the love and support that fills my heart with happy memories to this day.

For some moms, this is great; company is good. For other moms, they may be overstimulated, and the thought of entertaining company is just too much to handle in their lives. As a new mom, it's okay to set these boundaries with friends. And, as a visiting friend, asking what their needs are at that time is great to do before coming over for a visit. Decision making fatigue happens so much faster when someone is sleep deprived and juggling all of the stimulus input that comes with caring for a newborn. Asking "what do you need?" or "what can I do?" may be too much for someone to process and come up with a good answer. "Can I bring you lunch?" or "Can I pick you up any diapers or wipes when I run to the store?" may be more digestible questions and easier to answer.

A lot of people worry about germs, and rightly so. If they are good enough of a friend to drop by during this time of your life, then they are good enough of a friend to respect a "no holding the baby until you [the mama] are ready" decree.

At the very least, you can ask those filthy animals to wash their hands and keep their lips off your baby. The bottom line is that it's your baby and your boundaries.

I have heard all too often from patients and friends that they have a hard time with grandparents maintaining these set boundaries since they are family, such as the "no kissing" decree, and have even had people complaining to me in indignation that their relative who just gave birth won't let them see the baby until they get their whooping cough shot. My hot take on that is that any excuse they try to come up with to counter what the mama requests is a hot steaming pile of trash, and your friends and family members are not exempt from these boundaries if you set them. If they want to call you "unreasonable," that's on them, and they will (likely) get over it.

If you are comfortable with your scrubbed and sanitized friends and family holding the baby, they can snuggle them while you shower, eat a meal while it's still hot, or just lay horizontally on your couch, unencumbered by a small human for a little while.

Either way, the gesture of stopping by and the connection really helps with the isolated feeling, and it can lift spirits and make a new mom feel a little less overwhelmed.

BREASTFEEDING AND THE STRUGGLES OF FEEDING

There is a lot of stress that goes into managing the basic functions of keeping your child alive.

I'm not sure there was anything that I was less prepared
for when I became a mom than breastfeeding.

I really wanted that opportunity to bond with my baby and give them all of the immunity and benefits that came along with it. I put a lot of pressure on myself to be successful with it, and being perfectly honest, I went a little over the edge.

My first baby could not latch. I saw lactation consultants, went to "Milk Bar" (which was a super cool breastfeeding support group at the local women's hospital), got her lip and tongue tie fixed, and did all of the associated exercises. She just struggled with that latch, she was hungry, and she was small. Feeding her was critical to her survival. I was desperate to make it work. Calculating the time I was putting in, the effort was over 10 hours a day. Every two to three hours, I would attempt to feed her from each side, giving her a bottle when she would not latch, then pumping for 20 minutes to make more bottles and keep up my supply. By the time I finished the routine, it would be nearly time to start again. This went on 24 hours out of the day, every day, for weeks. It was challenging.

One day, at Milk Bar, the lactation consultant looked at me and said, "You have done literally everything you can to try and breastfeed this baby. Everyone in the community knows you because you have seen us all and tried it all. It is OKAY if you want to formula feed."

I needed to hear that. It still felt terrible, like I personally failed my baby by not being able to succeed in my attempts to just feed her, but once I let it go and switched over to formula, my stress level evaporated, allowing me to be more relaxed and happy. We also invested in a Baby Brezza, which is basically a formula Keurig, and let me tell you, if you're formula feeding, RUN—don't walk—to your local baby store and buy one. If that's the only tip you take from this book, it's life-changing.

My next kid had an awesome latch, but I just could not produce enough milk. Being a grizzled veteran of the insanity that came with the breastfeeding struggle the first time around, I was able to let that one go much more easily. Sometimes, you have to leverage your expectations against what is going to be best for everyone, and for me, that was allowing myself the grace to let it go and make sure both of my children were fed. The whole "breast is best" vs. "fed is best" argument is silly, especially in cases like mine, where my kids would have gone hungry without a logical intervention on my part.

The U.S. Dietary Guidelines for Americans 2020-2025, The American Academy of Pediatrics, and The World Health Organization all recommend and support exclusive breastfeeding for the first 6 months of your baby's life. According to a survey performed on breastfed babies born in 2019 by the CDC, only 24.9% of infants were exclusively breastfed up to 6 months. Some common issues reported that led to discontinuation of breastfeeding included poor latch of the baby, decreased lactation, unsupportive work, family or cultural environment, concerns about maternal medications, and concerns for the baby's overall weight gain and nutritional intake.

If you're having difficulty with breastfeeding and want to keep at it, some excellent resources include finding a lactation consultant or IBCLC in your area, reaching out to your local La Leche League, or joining a local breastfeeding support group.

No matter what you choose, just be kind to yourself. I admire women who work so hard to get the hang of breastfeeding and cheer them on during their wins in that season of their lives. But, if it's a colossal struggle for you, it's okay to save yourself the anguish I put myself through. You have nothing to blame yourself for if you can't make it work.

Both of my kids are beyond bottles now, and neither is holding a grudge against me for feeding them formula.

Grudges are reserved for giving them the wrong color cups and watering down the purple juice while hoping they don't notice (they always do).

I look back at the newborn period with a lot of fondness. Did I feel like I would never sleep again? Absolutely. Did I continue to be easily overwhelmed? Yup. Did I feel like I had been beaten up and was moving around a struggle? Abso-toot-a-lutely. Do I miss those sweet special moments with a tiny newborn snuggle bunny of a baby and that new baby smell? Every day. Once they got older and started to sleep through the night, I missed the quiet moments rocking them in the middle of the night when it felt like no other human was awake. When I was in the thick of it, I felt stressed and counted the moments until I could get back to sleep a lot of the time. Then, when I didn't need to get up with them anymore, I missed the extra time. With my second baby, I was prepared and continued to tell myself, "This won't last forever, and you will miss it when it's over." I have a sneaking suspicion that is going to be one of the main tenets of parenthood.

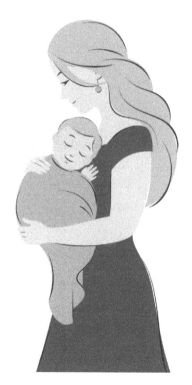

CHAPTER THREE:

Things aren't working like they are supposed to, and I hurt all over

The last two weeks of pregnancy are a really slow waddle to the finish. My back hurt every time I blinked, my pelvis felt like it was being held together by scotch tape, and one wrong move would result in a "mysterious" puddle. It was not wise to sit in a chair after me following a sneeze.

I could not wait for that sweet relief birth would bring and "have my body back to myself." Oh, what a fool I was.

Birthing and caring for a baby bring on different physical and mental challenges of their own, as we've discussed in previous chapters. For obvious reasons, I feel a lot of empathy with my postpartum patients and love working with them to try and navigate what is going on. I get so excited when I see a new mom on my schedule because we can do a lot to make her feel better in her body and provide her with some opportunities for self-care, and most of the time, I get to see the cute babies that come along to their appointments.

Regarding a postpartum mama's physical concerns, most commonly, I see lumbopelvic pain, pelvic floor dysfunction, diastasis recti, neck pain, and "Mommy's Thumb" (DeQuervain's tendonitis). So many factors go into why these conditions happen specifically in this population. We spoke briefly in chapter 1 about the rapid changes the body makes to accommodate growing a baby, we spoke of the effects of birthing the baby in chapter 2, and now we will talk about the fallout from those two factors, plus the body mechanics of holding our babies.

As a physical therapist, I am frequently extolling the value of taking care of your body and keeping yourself healthy and strong.

When we start to think about birth in its physical components, it is definitely similar to an injury that requires rehabilitation.

We are going to just dive right into the reasons why things aren't working as efficiently as they should and why they are possibly causing injuries and pain after the fact.

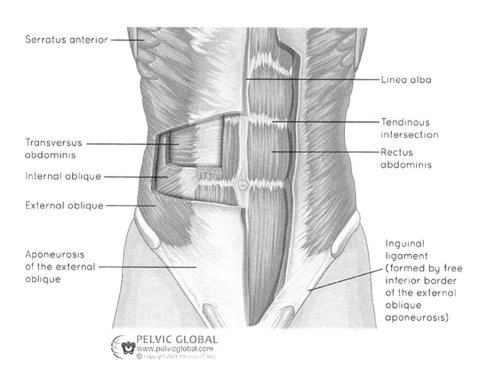

THE CORE

We hear a lot about "the core." Let's define what exactly that means The core consists of a 360-degree span of the muscles that surround your midsection. Anteriorly and laterally, we have the abdominals, which include the external obliques, the internal obliques, the rectus abdominis, and the transverse abdominis. Posteriorly and laterally, we have the gluteus maximus, the gluteus medius and minimus, the paraspinal group, and the multifidi muscles. A lot of the time, when people think "core," they are thinking of those six-pack muscles—the rectus abdominis. But we can see from the above list that the core is much more extensive than that.

A few functions of the core include stabilization of the spine and pelvis, support and protection of the abdominal organs, good posture, and intra-abdominal pressure management.

Structurally, when we become pregnant, the uterus grows, stretching and displacing the abdominal muscles. This will most often result in diastasis recti, which is a separation of the rectus abdominis through stretching the connective tissue that connects the two sides called the linea alba. Connective tissue is not contractile like a muscle, and therefore, after delivery, sometimes the linea alba has difficulty returning to its original form after that huge stretch. Think about stretching out a rubber band from both ends. The first time you stretch it, its going to return to normal fairly easily. The more and the farther you stretch this rubber band, the less likely it will be to return to normal.

Functionally, the implications of this can result in a dyssynergy of the abdominal muscles, weakness, and inefficient contraction of the abdominal group. If the abdominals are not working efficiently with the rest of the core group, we will see increased pain with abdominal contraction, increased low back pain from decreased anterior stability, over-recruitment of our posterior chain, and decreased intra-abdominal pressure management. This starts to give us some answers to questions like "Why does my back hurt?", "Why are my abdominal muscles still pooching out?", or "Why am I still sneeze-peeing?"

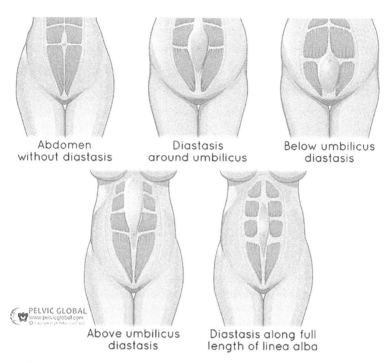

Abdomen without diastasis

Diastasis around umbilicus

Below umbilicus diastasis

Above umbilicus diastasis

Diastasis along full length of linea alba

Core weakness can lead to all the above issues and is why we often begin our skilled physical therapy sessions with neuromuscular re-education of appropriate abdominal contraction for efficient strengthening. Many times, I will be in clinic, and women will want to be performing difficult abdominal strengthening exercises to "get their abs back faster." I understand this temptation oh so well, but to make a dent in restoring an appropriate and healthy contraction, we must build back the foundation and start small, then build up from there. "Proximal stability before distal mobility," which is just a bunch of fancy pants words for "strong core, better movement overall." I will typically begin a new patient with diaphragmatic breathing with abdominal draw-ins, pelvic tilting, and braced marching, all demonstrated by the patient with good form. When good mastery is achieved, we progress to harder things. I have included three progressions of what these exercises look like in appendix A. When attempting these exercises, I will advise a patient or client to make sure they feel aware and connected to their movement and that they can move pain-free.

THE PELVIC FLOOR

Arguably, one could write a whole book about any of these conditions, but it is extra true for pelvic floor dysfunction following birth. I have so many patients come in with a referral from their OB/GYN telling me: "I didn't know that there was anything I could do to help with what I have going on." Well, I am here with my giant megaphone, shouting from the rooftops that there is help and you do not have to suffer in silence.

Sex shouldn't hurt, peeing while sneezing isn't your new normal, and you can have a life in which sitting for a long time does not make your tailbone feel like it is pulling.

For so many years, women have just accepted these things as the "status quo" after giving birth. Sex and bathroom talk was taboo or just not for polite conversation and company, but people are talking now and sharing their struggles with each other and, even better, their solutions that came when they received the help and care that they needed. Social media videos on TikTok and Instagram have been mostly informative and are raising awareness for the subject, too, despite some of the garbage one needs to sort through to find proper factual information. I am entertained by the accounts that have "Kegel dance classes," but I don't bop my pelvic floor to the beat of "La Cucaracha," nor do I recommend that you do so either until you have a good understanding of what healthy pelvic floor motion should feel like.

WHAT IS THE PELVIC FLOOR?

The pelvic floor is a group of muscles that lie in a sling-like fashion at the base of the pelvis and hold up the pelvic organs. I like to imagine them as a hammock for the bladder, uterus, and rectum. During pregnancy, the uterus becomes—ahem—a larger item for that hammock to hold up, and then vaginal delivery will cause intense stretching and sometimes injury to this area. So, it is no surprise that following birth, there is some work that often will need to be done to restore proper function to this muscle group.

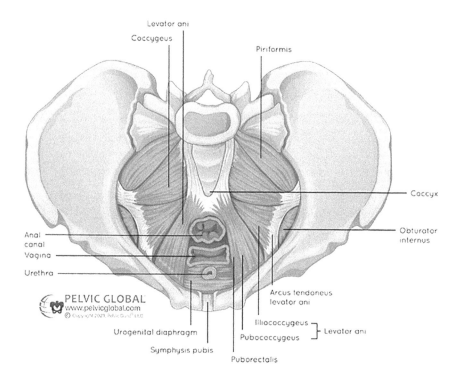

Often, postpartum patients will be referred to me at their 6- or 8-week visit with their OB. However, I also get a fair number of patients several years following the birth of their last child. Both types of patients do great with a good diagnosis and an appropriate plan of care. There is hope for all.

For the sake of not writing a 60,000-page book, I am going to group the types of pelvic floor issues into two main categories: overactive pelvic floor and underactive pelvic floor. There are many diverse categories of pelvic floor diagnoses and conditions within these two as well as overlap between the two, but I am going to just touch on the most commonly seen in our clinic.

Overactive pelvic floor conditions include dyspareunia (or pain with sexual intercourse), pain near the tailbone with sitting and other activities, a feeling of "ripping" or burning with bending down, leaking with impact activities, and/or unspecified hip and back pain.

Underactive pelvic floor conditions include urinary leakage and other types of incontinence, prolapse, and unspecified vaginal, hip, and back pain.

> *Has a well-meaning friend ever given you the advice, "Just do some Kegels; that's what helped me"? Even though it helped Becky with the good pelvic floor, it may not be right for everyone.*

As you can see above, a lot of the conditions that are caused by overactivity or underactivity are very similar. This is where I step on my "don't throw Kegels at everything" soap box.

To understand both overactive and underactive pelvic floors, we first need to understand pressure management of the intra-abdominal cavity. We've got our diaphragm up top, the pelvic floor at the bottom, and then the abdominals to manage the cylindrical intra-abdominal cavity. Picture these arranged around a can of soda.

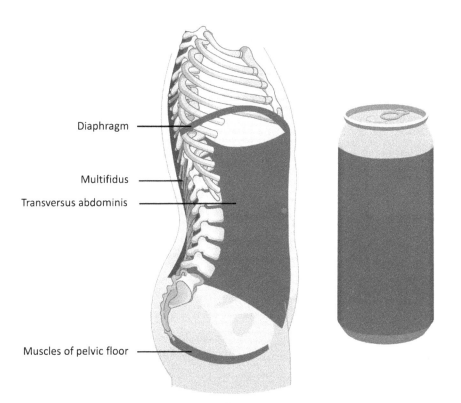

Diaphragm

Multifidus

Transversus abdominis

Muscles of pelvic floor

If there is a breach in one of the walls or the ceiling or floor of the can, you lose pressure. That dang breach is the cause of what makes us fear that unexpected sneeze in public.

In the postpartum state specifically, we are working against a lot of potential breaches in our cavity walls. In pregnancy, the baby pushes the diaphragm and organs upwards to the rib cage, decreasing the expansion of the lungs, ribs, and diaphragm; the uterus grows and separates the rectus abdominis in diastasis recti; and the pelvic floor must sustain larger and larger amounts of pressure and force. Postpartum, there is a great deal of carryover from these body changes that can affect the pelvic floor in a manner that causes overactivity or underactivity of the muscles and structures.

DYSPAREUNIA
Dyspareunia is the term for pain with sexual intercourse.

It can be caused by a variety of things and can occur during initial insertion or with deep penetration. After birthing a human that's the equivalent of a wrecking ball to our wonders down under, it may take some time for all of the equipment to be fully functional again. We see this condition a lot with overactive pelvic floors. However, underactive pelvic floors can cause it, too, via referred prolapse pain.

Overactivity and dyspareunia can be caused by scar tissue from the tearing sustained during childbirth. The scar tissue itself can cause pain in a variety of ways, but two notable things that will often happen are hypersensitivity at the scar site and muscle guarding around the area to "protect" the underlying structures. Many times, when patients have painful initial insertion during sexual intercourse or even tampon insertion, scar tissue is often the culprit.

In clinic, we will often teach our patients exercises called down training, which is relaxation of the pelvic floor as well as stretching of the associated muscle groups (i.e., hips, pelvic floor). We will discuss down training in further detail in the exercise portion of the book.

We can also perform manual stretching and scar work of the affected area to help tissue mobility and reduce muscle guarding. Manual work with introital (opening of the vagina) stretching looks a lot different than stretching a tight calf or hamstring. This particular technique involves an internal manual technique using one finger that stretches the tight pelvic floor muscles. We may even apply trigger point releases if any are present in the internal musculature. Often, when explaining the technique to a patient, I will tell them that just like we get trigger points in our shoulders, we can also develop them in the pelvic floor. The mechanics of the internal muscle release are very similar to how we release the trigger points from the outside of the body.

Another cause of pelvic floor muscle overactivity includes weakness of the core muscles. When the core is weak, intra-abdominal pressure is not being appropriately managed. The pelvic floor will sometimes overcompensate and work overtime for that core weakness. In addition to the above down training, this weakness is a great indicator as to why we retrain and strengthen the abdominals following birth. This will come up again when we talk about lower back and hip pain, as the core is so essential to a happy, harmoniously working body.

DYSPAREUNIA AND TRAUMA
Sometimes, when a traumatic birth occurs, dyspareunia follows.

Processing trauma in the brain is a very powerful and profound thing.

This will sometimes translate into non-specific pain and tightness of the pelvic floor. If you're a mother who is experiencing this, first off, I would like to say that I am sorry, I see you, and you are not alone. I wish I could give everyone suffering through that mental turmoil a hug. The birth of my first daughter became so scary so quickly, and I still sometimes have moments where I am terrified imagining the "what ifs." It took a lot of work and a lot of love for me to get to a place where I felt okay again. I encourage you to tap into your support system. Utilize all of the therapies! Physical therapy for your pelvic health and a counselor for your mental health and well-being. It's important to be open to the idea of acknowledging the situation and honoring it by doing what you can to take care of yourself and work through it.

Trauma may also include sexual assault, violence, or major traumatic events that are not related to childbirth or sex. We once had a patient who had severe dyspareunia following an extensive orthopedic surgery that left her so guarded and protective of her body that she was unconsciously creating so much tension in her pelvic floor muscles that it became too painful and scary for her to even use hygienic products. The body will do what it thinks it should to protect us from the effects of trauma.

Helping patients process trauma is not in our scope as physical therapists. If these patients are not currently being treated by a mental health professional, we are certainly going to start with recommending oneed or referring out for this. In therapy we will work on desensitization activities, progressive relaxation activities and diaphragmatic breathing, only progressing the patient to more invasive portions of the exam when they feel ready, and that it is in their comfort zone.

Just like any other diagnosis, we want to treat the whole person and lead them to the resources and professionals they need for success.

Dyspareunia can feel very daunting to the new mother, and can make it hard to connect to their spouse physically. After going through all of the literal labors of love involved with birthing, you deserve to be able to share love and intimacy with your partner without pain or restriction afterward. The prognosis for dyspareunia is so promising. I love seeing these patients walk through my door because I know they are going to feel a lot better pretty quickly. You absolutely do not have to suffer through this pain!

INCONTINENCE
"If peeing your pants is cool, call me Miles Davis." –Billy Madison

Oh, incontinence. I used to never wear anything but black workout pants to the gym in the event that excessive jumping would lead to a puddle. Once, I even suggested to my coach that he should put some newspaper down underneath my jump rope spot. Being a crazy, irreverent human with minimal shame, I did not mind making these jokes.

Some women come to me who are avoiding the gym altogether for fear this will happen to them. They deserve their self-care without having this fear!

With some good care to my pelvic floor function, I can now jump all over the place without a care in the world, and it's possible to help other women get there, too. We just need to get the word out that it's not so weird. In fact, about 47% of women report incontinence or leakage following the birth of a child. Are you sitting next to another mom? Cool. One of you probably has had leakage, if we are going straight off statistics, but more than likely, you've both had more than just a close call.

There are six types of incontinence that we currently have classifications for, and in this book, we will cover two of the most commonly seen postpartum: stress incontinence and urge incontinence.

In general, healthy urinary voiding guidelines include about 5-8 voids per day, every 2-4 hours.

It is recommended to drink half of your body weight in ounces of fluid per day, with about 65% of that being water.

For example, a 150-pound woman should aim to drink 75 ounces of fluid per day, 50 ounces or more being water. We ask a lot of questions about voiding: do you have painful urination? Can you fully empty your bladder? If you shift forward on the toilet, does more urine come out? Is your stream of urine strong and steady, or does it feel weak, spray, or start and stop mid-void? If you have difficulty with any of those mentioned items, you may find some help and relief with pelvic floor PT!

Stress incontinence occurs when there is urinary leakage with coughing, sneezing, jumping, lifting heavy objects, laughing, and other activities that cause an increase in intra-abdominal pressure. It is often seen in younger postpartum and athletic populations. Your bladder is located anteriorly in the pelvis on top of the pelvic diaphragm. Urine is stored in the bladder and exits the body through the urethra. The pelvic floor supports the bladder and the bladder sphincter. Pregnancy and childbirth can cause weakness from stretching and putting pressure on these structures (the 'smoosh' factor), which will reduce the ability to control urine output with increases in intra-abdominal pressure. The same can be said for a tight pelvic floor. With this tightness, shock and pressure are not appropriately distributed and can also cause leakage.

Once we determine the state of the pelvic floor, we can begin down training, stretching, and relaxation for the overactive pelvic floor and strengthening for the underactive pelvic floor. Following birth, a lot of women will tell me that they do not feel confident returning to the gym for fear of having an incident of leakage in public. As a big proponent of self-care for mamas, fill your cup, ladies. I want to be able to get women to the place where they feel comfortable doing whatever it is to get that cup up to the brim—without leaking over the top (ha!).

Urge incontinence is also referred to as "overactive bladder." As stress incontinence ties mainly to the issue of leakage, urge incontinence usually centers around increased frequency of urination. Many of these patients will have the urge to urinate and then have leakage before they even have a chance to make it to the restroom. Most of the time, these patients come in with the complaint of sudden leakage when they first get the urge to urinate, which results in increased urinary frequency. It creates a fear-based cycle of preventative measures to use the bathroom to avoid that leaking. They know where all the bathrooms are around town. Many times, their symptoms are associated with habits: "When I turn my key in the door when I get home, I have to get to the bathroom immediately or else I will have an accident." In these cases, pelvic floor strengthening can be indicated. In addition, a lot of the therapy includes something called "bladder retraining," where we keep a diary of bladder habits and find patterns that lead to increased frequency. We teach these patients pelvic floor and abdominal bracing to help control and reduce the leakage with the urge. These patients will typically try and limit their water intake because they are afraid of needing a bathroom. We try and discourage them from doing so. We like to give the goal of increasing the time between voids instead.

Other treatments of incontinence can include the use of biofeedback or electric stimulation to help retrain the pelvic floor muscles to contract properly, medications like overactive bladder agents, or placement of a pessary. A pessary is a device that gives support to the vaginal walls to help hold up the bladder better. Pessaries are also often utilized in the presence of prolapse.

I get it. Peeing your pants as an adult can be humiliating, and the stress of worrying about that is something you don't need to deal with.

Instead of writing to Pampers headquarters for a two-for-one package of baby and adult diapers, there are a lot of things you can try to reduce your incidents of leakage and increased frequency and get back to jumping around and living the dry life.

PROLAPSE

Prolapse is a condition where there is decreased support of the pelvic organs, causing them to descend into the vaginal wall. Women will often tell me that they feel like their pelvic floor is "heavy," feels like it's "falling," or that there is a lot of downward pressure. Sometimes, I will hear that they have difficulty completing a bowel movement and need to place a finger in the vaginal cavity in order to provide support in order to be able to complete their bowel movement (often called "splinting"). Otherwise, they feel like they cannot fully empty while voiding.

Prolapse is very common in postpartum women, especially following vaginal delivery. In a study published in the International Urogynecology Journal, up to 90% of postpartum women had certain types of prolapse present on exam. Additionally, following the first vaginal delivery, a woman is four times more likely to have a prolapse diagnosis which jumps to being over eight times more likely following a second vaginal delivery. That is a very high incidence to consider. Sometimes, prolapse will be asymptomatic. However, other times, symptoms can appear with urinary and bowel voids (weakened streams, difficulty fully emptying); pain with sex or difficulty reaching orgasm; lower back pain; abdominal pressure; and/or pressure, pain, or heaviness in the vagina and the perineum.

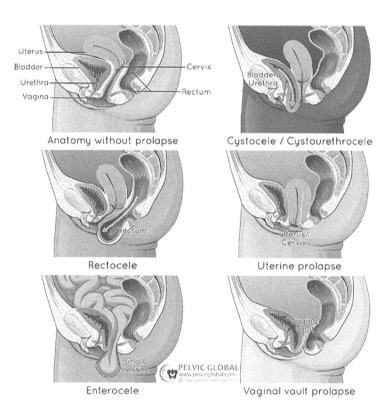

Anatomy without prolapse

Cystocele / Cystourethrocele

Rectocele

Uterine prolapse

Enterocele

Vaginal vault prolapse

There are different severities and classifications of prolapse, and they are named for the organ that is drooping out of place. Depending on these factors, treatment will vary. Strengthening of the hips, core, and pelvic floor may be indicated and may be very successful in reducing the prolapse. Instruction in body mechanics and appropriate muscle bracing with increasing the abdominal pressure to reduce the downward pressure on the pelvic diaphragm is also helpful. In more severe cases and cases that do not respond well to conservative management, a device called a pessary can be inserted into the vagina. A good way to think of how this device functions is to consider it a "space saver." It will help provide support to the vaginal walls to keep the prolapsing organ in place. Surgery to place a pelvic or bladder mesh can be indicated in severe cases as well.

> *Prolapse is a diagnosis that comes with a lot of fear surrounding it, but I am here to reassure you that it is very manageable with awareness and some changes to the way we think about our posture and our core engagement.*

Learning "The Knack"- a technique where we contract our abdominals and pelvic floor before a sneeze, cough or lifting a heavy load will go a very long way in mitigating that downward pressure on the pelvic floor. If this is something that you are diagnosed with, don't panic. Educate yourself on what you can do to manage that pressure and making more pelvic floor more efficient.

PUDENDAL NEURALGIA

Pudendal neuralgia can occur during a vaginal delivery, usually in the later stages of labor, as the baby passes through the pelvis and past the pudendal nerve. This nerve supplies sensation to the labia, clitoris, vulva, perineum, and anus and allows the sphincters of the anus and bladder to contract and relax. Patients will usually describe this as a burning or itching pain. Sitting makes those symptoms feel worse, and sometimes, even the feel of clothes on the skin will make the area feel uncomfortable. Occasionally, people will note that sitting on a toilet will make the pain feel better temporarily, but sitting on a regular chair or bike seat for any length of time will make it feel worse. Some people note bowel or bladder dysfunction secondary to the nerve's role in controlling the sphincters as well.

Typically, when this injury occurs, exercises and manual therapy for relaxation of the pelvic floor muscles can help if this tightness is causing entrapment and irritation of the nerve.

LOWER BACK PAIN AND SACROILIAC JOINT DYSFUNCTION
Pregnancy is a heck of a journey for the lower back and pelvis. They are the real MVPs of that wild ride.

It's very common to have lower back and pelvic pain throughout the duration of the prenatal period. Following delivery, there are a lot of reasons for lower back pain to persist. Ligamentous changes continue beyond birth as the hormone relaxin stays in the body. This will persist even longer with breastfeeding mothers. Relaxin will cause the joints to stay looser and less stable, and although the looser ligaments may not be causing pain, the lack of dynamic muscle support and function to support those joints may become an issue.

The spine and the pelvis like to be stable; otherwise, pain and tomfoolery will ensue. However, they also need to be able to move—we aren't walking around all stiff like robots at any point of the day! The lumbar spine relies more on dynamic stability, like the muscular strength of the abdominals, hips, and paraspinals. This stability is more fluid and changes to allow for movement and articulation of the lumbar vertebra. We want these structures to move well. However, the sacroiliac joint relies more on the static stability of ligaments and is not supposed to move.

The lower back will be used a lot more with picking up a baby regularly. At times, it can be hard to have the perfect body and lifting mechanics when the twenty-pound object you're picking up is squirming and trying to do a double backflip out of your arms. So, there are a few factors—despite how cute they are—that are working against you in this department. Add to that the fact that your core has been severely compromised and is likely weak and lacking the ability to contract efficiently to manage spinal stability with movement, and it's the perfect storm for injury.

Pregnancy habitus, or the changes in your body's shape and posture during pregnancy, will cause an overload on the body's ability to support itself and result in weakness in the abdominals and outer hips. It brings the lower back into increased extension (lordosis). The belly pulls forward and sways the back forward. The bump grows outward, and the outer and inner hips become weaker and less efficient. This associated weakness will carry over to the postpartum period. All of those structures just described will—you guessed it—give support to the spine and pelvis. The dynamic stability previously mentioned is comprised of these muscle groups. When they are compromised, it can create a vulnerable situation for the lower back and SI joints, making them more susceptible to injury or pain.

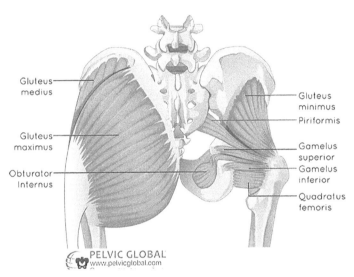

In a typical postpartum lower back pain patient, we want to strengthen the hips and core in a manner that does not overload the muscles or allow larger muscles like the hip flexors to compensate. Exercises like the dead bug, brace marching, and side-lying clamshells are great for this. In most back patients, the body is very good at giving us warning signals to indicate that something is painful. For example, someone with a herniated disc may have pain with sitting or bending the spine forward, and someone with an SI joint issue may have more of an issue with extending back through the spine, getting in and out of bed, or otherwise changing positions. We have to be mindful to move in a way that helps strengthen and stabilize the spine without further injuring the involved area.

When it comes to treating these conditions, there is a little more that goes into the clinical decision-making and coming to an accurate diagnosis, which is why I highly recommend seeing a physical therapist who is familiar with not only back pain but also treating it in a postpartum demographic.

NECK PAIN, UPPER BACK PAIN, AND MOMMY'S THUMB

This cluster of postpartum pain and conditions can be easily blamed on carrying our babies around. Those little barnacles just destroy anything resembling good posture, and we are all just walking around like slump-a-mumps as a result. With breastfeeding and cradling our babies, we have the natural inclination to protect and wrap our arms around them, causing our shoulders to round forward and our heads to lean down and in towards our little ones. This will put some increased stress and stretch on the posterior structures.

This is going to result in a few different issues.

In the upper neck, this is going to cause a lot of posterior stress, which can give you a stiff neck or even cause a herniated disk to occur.

In the upper back, the muscles that pull your scapula together will be stretched and become weak. When these muscles are weak, they won't support the spine or shoulder girdle as well, which is going to cause the mid-back vertebra to get tight to compensate for the lack of muscle stability and be why you may feel like you need someone to give you a good back cracking.

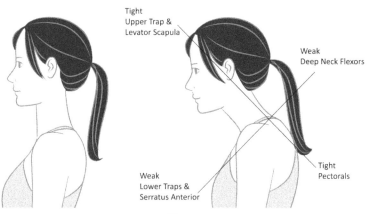

The main treatments that we are going to use for this cluster of diagnoses will be postural re-education and stretngthening our neck and postural muscles. Postural re-education includes things like making workstations more ergonomic and utilizing good postures when breastfeeding. It can be very hard to breast feed and find the ideal position for your baby to latch, however for mom, we recommend trying to sit upright with your feet on a stool to elevate baby and keep your trunk and head more upright. Sidelying is also a great option because it will allow you to support and prop your head on a pillow.

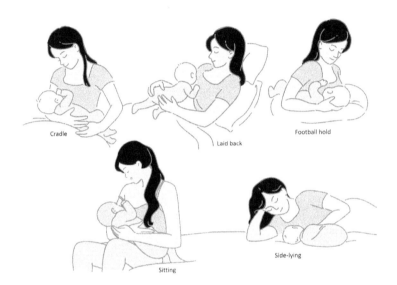

Cradle

Laid back

Football hold

Sitting

Side-lying

MOMMY'S THUMB (DE QUERVAIN'S TENOSYNOVITIS)

My second baby is a stage five clinger. That little nugget wanted all the snuggles all of the time. Since I am right-handed, I was holding her primarily on my left side, her head crooked in my elbow and my hand tucked up under her bottom for support. When I would finally sleep, I would wake up, and my wrist would be burning.

De Quervain's is an 'overuse' syndrome of the tendons of the thumb.

The constant load (the lazy baby loaf) on the tendons can cause them to become inflamed and swollen. Without proper rest and reduction of that inflammation, this condition is very likely to continue in a pain loop cycle. However, you can attempt to strengthen and stretch the areas around the inflamed tendons and then eventually apply strengthening and stretching to the thumb tendons as they become less painful. Postural re-education and encouraging feeding the baby while holding them in the other arm can be helpful, too. However, I have had many conversations with many moms of new babies who have a "side" they've come to prefer and refuse to feed being held on the opposite side. Icing this area for about 15 minutes two to three times per day can also be helpful in reducing inflammation and pain in this area.

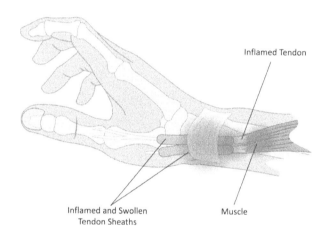

Inflamed Tendon

Inflamed and Swollen
Tendon Sheaths

Muscle

OTHER MATERNAL ISSUES WITH BIRTH

There are multiple other issues that can occur with childbirth. I was selective with the above-chosen conditions to try and be inclusive of a large variety of orthopedic and pelvic health common postpartum issues.

I see a lot of fear and the idea that this population is fragile. That has to change. As women, we are so resilient, and our bodies are capable of so much.

There is nothing to be afraid of if you are having issues postpartum. Take a deep breath, and make a plan. Reach out for help.

My bottom line here is that there is help for whatever is going on, you are not alone, and I encourage you to find the supporting resources to lead you to wellness. There is no special award or merit badge for bearing pain that you do not need to live with. I know that time is limited when you have little ones, and it is so easy to put yourself on the back burner. However, your health is important, and these things can get worse over time if you ignore them. I used to be the "ignore it until it goes away" gal—if I were a car, I'd be riding around with the check engine light on. A car broken down on the side of the road is not doing anyone any favors, though. Eventually, it catches up, making the road back to wellness an even longer one.

CHAPTER FOUR:

When is it safe to go back to the gym?

Once upon a time, a very well-meaning male fitness professional asked me, "When can you start working out again after having a baby without having to worry about your vagina falling out?"

At first, it's easy to laugh at this question and give him a hard time. But, if we are being perfectly honest, a lot of us have probably wondered the same thing postpartum, and good on that guy for wanting to know in order to be able to help serve his female clientele!

There are so many variables when it comes to returning to fitness. What kind of birth did you have? What type of fitness or athletics are you trying to return to? What was your level of activity prior to getting pregnant? What about prior to birth?

A lot of women get the "all clear" at their 6- to 8-week visit with the OB/GYN, but what if you want to return to higher-level, competitive sports?

It's unlikely that you're going to feel safe and comfortable running a marathon or deadlifting over 250 pounds at just six weeks postpartum, and most likely, you REALLY should not feel safe and comfortable doing either of those things at six weeks postpartum! So then, where do we draw the line?

Immediately following birth, we know that we are going to have to be able to move around, pick up our infant, and within a few days, pick up their car seat. (This will be two weeks out in the case of a c-section). If you have a toddler, there will be a 30-pound "object" you may be lifting regularly as well, but it's not likely that you are going to be doing full-on bike sprints or even feeling like this would be an option.

I am going to bring back the analogy from earlier about birth being like recovering from an injury or surgery.

Just as you would not want to rush your recovery following an ACL repair or a muscle tear, you do not want to rush to return to sports and exercise following birth, whether you had a vaginal birth or a cesarean section—the key word here being "rush." Following surgery or an injury, there's a period of time for healing in which one needs to follow a timeline or protocol. Depending on what took place, you will often be able to identify certain activities that are safe and beneficial during different portions of the recovery period.

If your friend had her rotator cuff repaired and then the next day asked you to go play tennis, you would very likely tell Gina to slow her roll and let herself recover for a bit.

I personally think the same concept can be easily applied to the postpartum period, and I've devised some loose guidelines to help the mama athlete get back to training. As with anything, this is an example and not a guide supported by empirical evidence. Make sure that you consult with your OB and your local physical therapist to make sure that certain levels of activity are appropriate and safe for you!

With everything, there is a spectrum of variables that we need to consider. If you were working out recreationally up until birth, your recovery following birth is likely going to go more smoothly. If you were an elite athlete and worked on training to a high capacity until delivery, that sliding scale will be different as well.

BIRTH TO TWO WEEKS

From birth to two weeks, your main precautions will include avoiding activity that increases pain, pelvic pressure, or incontinence or that increases the difficulty you have controlling the passing of gas. Additionally, with a c-section, there will be no lifting of anything heavier than your baby, no reaching overhead, and no twisting of your trunk area.

There has been some talk on social media about the placenta leaving a dinner plate-size wound behind. This is great to be mindful of during this period of your recovery. The great thing is that the wound is going to get smaller and smaller by the day and likely be healed around the one-week mark. The body is incredible.

No matter what kind of birth you had, walking as much as tolerable as soon as your legs are working again is highly recommended. Get up, get behind that hospital baby bassinet, and push your sweet little bundle of joy around the Labor and Delivery hallways. Feel free to proclaim how cute your baby is, how cute the other babies are that parents are proudly parading down the halls, and how much of a bad mama-jamma you are for bringing life into the world. Rock that post-birth waddle swagger as far as you can manage until you start to feel any pain or fatigue. You absolutely do not want to push into painful parameters!

Deep belly breathing, called diaphragmatic breathing, is also indicated at this time. All of your organs were just smushed up into your rib cage and pelvis. If you had a c-section, things in there were batted around all willy-nilly, too. You want to start to expand that intra-abdominal cavity and get things moving and settling properly.

Ankle pumps are excellent to perform to help with any postpartum swelling you may have, to prevent blood clots, and to strengthen the ankles.

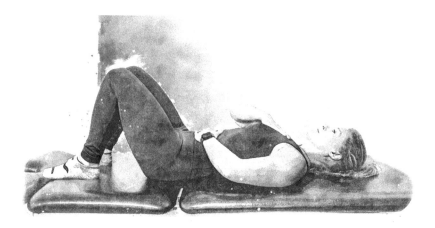

Kegels can be performed almost immediately following birth unless you've had a grade 3 or 4 perineal tear. In that case, you'll want to wait until weeks 3 or 4 or until you receive clearance from your OB. Starting to engage the pelvic floor will not only help with recovery but will also strengthen one of your most important pressure management muscles, which will help with all efficiency of movement. (Don't forget from our earlier section on the pelvic floor that not all Kegels are created equal! We want to make sure we can also relax the pelvic floor.)

Shoulder rolls and pinches can be performed almost immediately postpartum to help with the postural discomforts of holding your baby and breastfeeding.

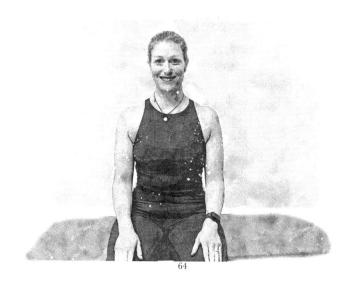

WEEKS TWO TO FOUR

In weeks two to four postpartum, you can start to move and strengthen your body a little more. Precautions stay about the same in general: nothing to increase pelvic pressure or pain, being aware and able to control bowel and bladder activities and the passage of gas, and nothing to increase the abdominal pain from a c-section.

As both a mom and physical therapist, I like to add some standing strengthening exercises, like heel raises, standing hip abductions, standing marches, etc. This is a great way to start functionally activating the abdominals and strengthening the hips.

I also like to add in some quadruped work and spinal movement, such as cat camels and abdominal draw-ins, in this position. I love getting in different positions with exercise as soon as possible because it allows us to play with how our muscles work with or against gravity and allows us to access muscle contractions differently. In short, it makes our muscles smarter and more efficient with how they contract.

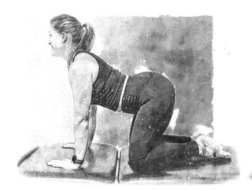 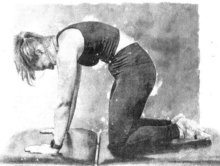

Around week two is when I recommend starting the posterior pelvic tilt series in postpartum PT. This is the foundational movement of the diastasis repair series and is a nice, gentle strengthener that is safe and efficient. There are so many ways to progress and add on to the posterior pelvic tilt, and leading up to this two-week period, mastering the basics is an excellent way to start to feel those abdominals working and bracing again.

As far as walking is concerned, you can go for longer distances and brisker paces, and you can also start doing other cardio like riding a stationary bike if it is not painful on your perineum. You should also still be doing your postural strengthening exercises and Kegels.

Some people like to go back to the gym at this time for the social aspect and the support of seeing their friends. I have no issues with this in the two- to four-week period as long as mom is making smart decisions. As we talked about above, just living and caring for your family is going to be a lot of physical work.

Your lady parts are not going to explode if you go to the gym and ride the bike and do some bird dogs with your friends, but you do need to be sure to pace yourself and not over-exert yourself if you're not feeling up to par just yet.

In fact, some research supports a safe return to moderate exercise between the two- to six-week marks. In a study by Nygaard et al, early exercise intervention was either helpful or not harmful to pelvic health. We already know that exercising helps with many physical and mental variables, so having this information helps to dispel some of the fear and apprehension people have during the postpartum period.

WEEKS FOUR TO SIX
During weeks four to six, you can start adding more focused and functional strength exercises.

Now, you can add a side-lying series for hip strengthening, such as clamshells or hip abductions, since the lateral muscles of the body often become weak during pregnancy. Anyone who knows me as a PT knows that I love a good application of a clamshell series. This is good for so many things, especially with strengthening muscles that will help to dynamically stabilize the core and spine.

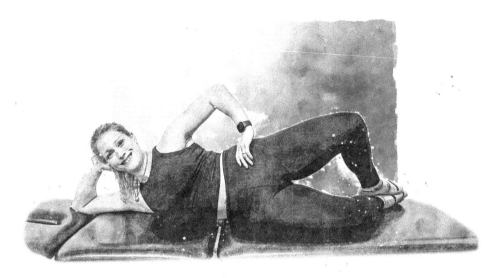

Quadruped work is useful for core re-education, too. You can make this more difficult by adding arm and leg reaches to also challenge and strengthen pelvic stability. Heaven knows that that pelvis worked overtime with a capital "O" that whole pregnancy. Be nice to it.

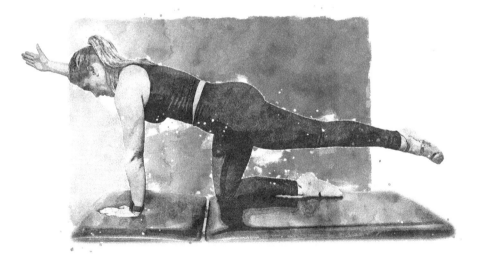

Progressing the pelvic tilt series to tabletop holds with a demonstration of good, safe form is also indicated around this time. I like to do tabletop tap-downs with good lumbopelvic stability and no pain in the abdominals around this time as well. These are like my daily vitamin exercise for the postpartum patient and especially the postpartum athlete. (However, hold off on this until 6 to 8 weeks if you've had a c-section.)

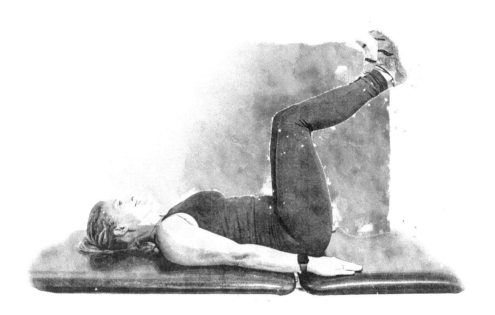

As you start to increase your intensity with strengthening the abdominals, you'll want to be mindful that you are not straining and that you are able to brace your core throughout the duration of the exercise. I still like to keep the core and spine mostly neutral and perform gentle stabilization exercises from there.

It's at weeks 6-8 that you are able to start adding in squats and lunges with good form and abdominal activation in the absence of pelvic floor pain or pressure. In a normal vaginal birth, you can start to integrate more exercises closer to returning to sport. You can start to very gradually increase lighter impact activities without loss of control of your bowels or bladder. Pull-ups with control of your core may be performed without pain. You can start to increase abdominal strengthening with the same precautions as previously noted. This is a great time period to start to discuss squatting safely with a load when postpartum. Squatting will naturally cause the pelvic floor to become active, meaning it is going to need to be ready and willing to work. In order to safely return to building the squat back up, you need to be able to demonstrate good efficiency in intra-abdominal pressure (IAP) management. I see a lot of lumbar faults at the bottom of the squat in the postpartum athlete leading to lower back injuries from core insufficiency and poor management of IAP. Air squats or box squats while holding a good abdominal brace (transverse abdominis contraction) is an excellent exercise to master before loading any weight on any barbells.

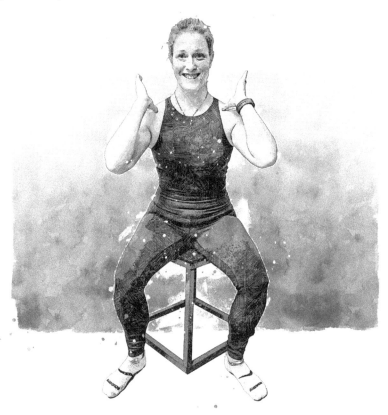

WEEK 8 AND BEYOND

During weeks 8 through 12, you can start adding increased resistance to your heavy strengthening work, and you can introduce higher-impact running and jumping closer to week 12. You'll want to be mindful of bladder control as you increase impact. At this point, you want to be aware of occasional leakage and/or a feeling of heaviness in the pelvic floor and report back to your OB in case it might indicate the need for a pelvic health evaluation by a qualified physical therapist.

For athletes that regularly participate in higher-impact sports or activities, a pelvic health exam may be wise to rule out the presence of a more moderate prolapse before increasing the volume and frequency of the activity.

The postpartum athlete will be more likely to have leakage with heavier lifting and higher-impact activities. It is good to be mindful of this and to use it as a metric for improving the quality of movement as well as breath and core control in order to perform these activities without leakage.

By 12 weeks, you can mostly be at the baseline of your sport and progress as tolerated.

Your main precautions are avoiding putting too much stress and strain on the pelvic floor and avoiding causing abdominal strain and lower back injury secondary to weakness of the abdominals.

This is generally the same for both vaginal and cesarean births at this particular week postpartum. With c-sections, I tend to advise smart decisions along with good mobility when stretching the abdominals. I think there is a need for this mobility post-op, but due to the surgical repair of these anterior structures, they can be a little stiff and often hypersensitive. I give extension-based exercises to tolerance in order to improve the scar mobility with functional movement.

There is a lot to be gained with progressively loading and increasing variables at this point. With lifting, being able to efficiently control the motion as well as brace the core and pelvic floor will be valuable. Making smart decisions about what your body can handle and adapt to will be crucial around this point. Many will state that they are starting to get impatient with their progress and want to speed it up. This is where we see the highest rate of postpartum injury, whether they be orthopedic or pelvic floor-related.

Finding the line between trusting your body and
challenging it just enough is going to be the sweet spot at
12 weeks and beyond.

Don't move on to the next harder thing until you've mastered your progression. It's time to clean things up and make your form look solid.

A NOTE ON RETURNING TO RUNNING

Additional research and criteria have been provided for returning to running in the postpartum patient. The Journal of Women's Pelvic Health published an article in June of 2022 stating that the timeline to return to running is a little more fluid depending on several biomechanical, musculoskeletal, and pelvic health conditions being met (Christopher et al.). They present and include in this article the "Run Readiness Scale" (Payne et al.), which asks questions about pelvic and abdominal health (control of urine and feces), impact readiness, and the ability to demonstrate good muscular endurance (ability to perform single leg calf raises, single leg bridging) and proper running gait (hip and knee strength and position, knees being stiff and step rates), as well as physiological factors such as sleep and nutritional quality, cardiovascular health (BP, risk of blood clot), and infection risk.

They provide a nice decision-making tree that walks the patient through ascending criteria before moving on to the next phase. It begins with the ability to walk 30 minutes without any pelvic floor heaviness or bladder leakage, then progressing to a walk/run over a shorter distance, and then increasing volume incrementally until the patient is back to running without symptoms. It's important to note that injury risk also includes a host of orthopedic injuries associated with running, secondary to the decreased strength of the core and hip muscles that are prevalent postpartum. Setting a goal that increases either intensity or volume and not both at once is a good strategy to not overdo it too quickly, and it helps control variables a little more closely. For example, if someone increases their distance by a quarter mile successfully this week, I would suggest they hold off on intensity or speed increases.

For me, each time I came back from birth, I used the postpartum period to relearn the basics and work on the fundamentals of good form.

It was so easy to get in my own head and compare "old Lauren" to this "new Lauren" who was not as strong or as fast.

Once I started looking at this period as an opportunity to rebuild from scratch, I was able to be more patient with myself. I was able to put in that well-needed work to become more efficient and cleaner with my lifting form, gymnastics form, running form, etc. I am not the same athlete as I was before giving birth, but I am also not even close to being the same person.

When I did get in my own head, it was all fear-based. "What if I'm not good enough anymore?" Holy cats! If a friend told me that, I would first hug them and then tell them that they are insane and they are SO MUCH BETTER than before. We cannot measure ourselves with the same metrics as before because our bodies have been pushed to their limits much further than before. Just as I encourage my friends to love themselves fully in this season of their lives, I also encourage myself to do the same.

I know we talked about this handy dandy return-to-sport timeline, yet it only goes up to 12 weeks. I want to take a moment to mention that I did not feel 100% at 12 weeks postpartum. Not even close. I didn't feel 100% at six months or nine months postpartum, either. I think, on average, with both pregnancies, it took me at least a year to start feeling like my body was working without the asterisk of those self-limiting beliefs that I mostly placed on myself. With both pregnancies, I had expectations of being 100% sooner than a year after giving birth. My second baby was an end-of-June baby, and I had dreams of wearing a bikini and looking fly by August. I applaud pregnant Lauren for her optimism. We all need that glass-half-full vibe in our lives, but wow. Expectations vs. reality were divergent, and I am okay with that. FYI, I still wore the bikini because I am, in fact, fly 'til I die, no matter what my body looks like.

BENEFITS OF WORKING OUT POSTPARTUM

What if exercise was not really your thing prior to getting pregnant, and you are wanting to become more active now? I love this! High five! There are so many benefits of postpartum exercise. I am a huge proponent of the promotion of exercise for the improvement of general health and wellness.

Research supports a wide range of physical and mental benefits of exercising postpartum.

Exercise can help with improvement in aerobic capacity (improvement with carrying an infant while doing 100 other things), improvement in bone density (to fight the potential effects of lactation), improvement in mood (goodbye to Momzilla!), decreasing anxiety and depression, decreasing obesity, and can also result in an increased likelihood of your children wanting to be healthier and more active.

So, not only are you doing good things for your own health, your example is proven by research to have a positive influence on your kids, too. That's a great reason in itself! If you want your kids to live it and do it, be it!

Being a parent is so rewarding, but it can be hard. If you have a recreational or exercise activity that you love doing and that helps you to fill your cup, this is your reminder to use it to breathe joy and happiness into your life. This is your reminder to use it to show your babies that you are strong and that prioritizing your health is important. This is your reminder to be grateful for a body that not only can make life but can move and be capable of great things.

If you're like me and sometimes that voice in your head tells you that "It won't be good enough," try and focus on the joy of just doing it, absent of criticism.

We deserve to move with joy. And to also maybe have 45 minutes to an hour away from our kids to decompress.

STRATEGIES FOR GETTING A WORKOUT IN WITH KIDS

Something that I really like to brainstorm for myself and others is accessibility to fitness with managing child care.

I was (am) one of those moms that is way more worried in my head about my kids bothering other people at the gym, so much so that it is really hard for me to relax and enjoy the workout if they are there. I love the idea of them seeing us work out and setting healthy examples for them, but I also worry that they will burn down the gym or lead an uprising from the children's room at my friend's CrossFit gym.

I wish I could be more like the parents who seamlessly work out while their kids behave off to the side. My children are wild animals despite my best efforts for public domestication, albeit cute wild animals.

What works best for me right now is building workouts into the day while they are at school, over my lunch break, or prior to pick-up.

Another thing I like to do as an early bird is get up and work out before they even wake up. I was able to buy a cheap spin bike and some small exercise equipment, so I can get a workout in before the onset of the day when the little ones start asking for their eggies and purple juice. I usually go to bed pretty early (read: I am boring at parties) in order to get up early, but it's amazing how much I get done in those quiet morning hours (for example, writing this book).

Some gyms have childcare, and there are a lot of "mom fit"/stroller classes out there. Strap those kiddos into your jogging stroller and go nuts. These places are great for meeting other like-minded parents and expanding your social circle of parent friends, too!

> *The bottom line of this section is that there are so many ways to get a workout in—somehow—that works with your life.*

It's easy to make excuses—I've made them all. We are tired and busy, and the days are too short. I will suggest to patients to start small. Make a commitment to yourself to get 10-15 minutes of exercise per day for 30 days, then increase the time until you're happy with it. The 10- to 15-minute commitment is a small, digestible amount of time that someone will be likely to stick to. Do it when they nap, right before they get up, after they go to bed, or over your lunch break when they are at school or daycare. You can schedule that time without even having to make special arrangements. Start simple and with something you really like so that you will be more likely to stick to it.

You are worth investing the time in yourself, and you're going to need to keep up your strength for when your kid is a toddler who will challenge your ability to move fast to prevent them from running away from you in public at top speeds and climbing up the furniture at your in-laws to attempt to throw the good china off the top shelf.

CHAPTER FIVE:

I'm hungry

Growing a baby is like housing a parasitic vampire that is leeching all of your nutrients and energy. Again, can't give us mamas enough credit for that massive job.

After the big event, we can feel pretty drained.

Energy is hard to come by thanks to the recovery your body needs as well as the whole not sleeping thing. There is discomfort at the baby's point of exit, and you are now lugging around your newly-outside barnacle, aka your tiny human. This makes it naturally hard to come by any rest.

Feeding your body for recovery and sustaining enough energy for the day-to-day is going to be crucial for getting by, even more so if you are breastfeeding.

After having both of my children, I had a lot of trouble sitting down to eat. I was all over the place and felt rushed most moments of the day. Tiny humans were my priority, and I did not give myself time or grace to eat. Something that eventually worked for me was setting up a snack bucket next to the nursery chair. I included high-density snacks like nuts, granola, and dried fruit, and in the overnight hours that I spent rocking my girls, I would snack on different healthy but easy-to-eat foods (think one-handed foods and not super loud to chew). This at least allowed me to get in some controlled calories and not defer to just skipping eating to get something else done. Other mothers have told me some tips they found helpful, such as prepping convenient mini meals like chicken and rice or oatmeal and making smoothies (another one-handed meal for the win!).

General postpartum nutrition guidelines are similar to the nutrition guidelines for while you are pregnant. The better the food you put into your body, the better the health outcomes and quality of energy. Choose foods that are natural and nutrient-dense, such as lean meats and veggies. Throw in some high-quality carbohydrates like sweet potatoes and brown rice. If you are breastfeeding, you want to aim to have 330-400 calories more than usual. The hard part to discern is what "the usual" is. This is going to be determined by body weight, activity level, and your body's basic needs for energy.

> *The better quality of food you eat, the better the energy you will have. Take it from a girl who tried to live on caffeine and a dream—you are going to want to feed yourself so that you can thrive!*

I am no nutritionist, but I can definitely tell you that cold brew does not make a sufficient lunch.

NUTRITION CONSIDERATIONS FOR THE BREASTFEEDING MOTHER

We have already spoken a bit about breastfeeding mothers needing 330 to 400 calories more per day than non-breastfeeding mothers to help meet the demands of the energy required for lactation, your body's process to produce milk from your mammary glands.

Many of my breastfeeding patients report that they stay pretty hungry throughout the day, so getting those 330-400 calories is not a problem.

Others have a little more trouble getting food down. I've seen it go both ways! Setting yourself up to get enough food throughout the day to meet your body's needs is going to be really important for this time in your life. A lot of times, breastfeeding moms will notice their supply drop significantly if they are not eating enough. It is important to find the balance your body needs.

HOW TO DECIDE WHAT TO EAT AND WHY

Protein, carbohydrates, and fats are what we call macronutrients, and these make up the bulk of our caloric intake. These are the more popular categories that people focus on when talking about nutrition. We hear and see marketing for "low-fat" or "low-carb, keto, sugar-free," etc. Some people track "their macros" and are referring to these three food groupings. I don't have good recommendations for an ideal macro split as it will differ from person to person with their nutritional needs and goals in the postpartum period, but I can run you through why these macronutrients each shine in their own way for the postpartum mother.

Carbohydrates are essential for energy.

They literally fuel the mitochondria of our cells to make adenosine triphosphate (ATP), our biological source of cellular energy. They are also delicious.

Protein helps with cellular regeneration and recovery of cells, especially muscle tissue, which is important as our bodies heal from birth.

It also helps us to feel fuller longer and provides immunity support. Getting around 25-30 grams of protein per meal is a great building block for setting up what your meals throughout the day are going to look like. About 70-100 grams of protein per day are recommended when pregnant and breastfeeding, and then that number goes up to 100-120g of protein per day for the athlete mama. My husband makes fun of my obsession with protein for myself and the kids, but it has so many health benefits!

Fat helps with hormone regulation—most notably estrogen
and progesterone.

When you look at the macronutrients in this light, it is clear that each plays an important role in our day-to-day wellness as healing mothers. It is important to choose high-quality and healthy versions of these macronutrients. If you have trouble making a decision, think of choosing things as close as possible to their natural form so that you avoid highly processed food. Avoiding added sugar, processed materials, and trans fats is typically a good game plan.

We have an increased need for certain micronutrients, especially calcium and iron. It is also recommended to continue taking a prenatal vitamin to get important vitamins and nutrients.

Our bodies secrete calcium into the breast milk for our babies, and our bodies need to replenish those stores for ourselves. An average consumption of 1000 mg of calcium per day is recommended. A glass of milk has about 300 mg of calcium. Dark, leafy greens, as well as almonds, are also foods high in calcium.

Iron is very important for breastfeeding mothers and improving energy levels in general. Iron helps to produce hemoglobin in our red blood cells. Hemoglobin helps to carry oxygen from the lungs in the bloodstream, which is essential for creating our energy on the cellular level in the form of ATP. Low iron can result in anemia. Dark leafy greens make an appearance here again as a good source of iron. We also find iron in lean meats and most cereals. During pregnancy, 22-23 mg of iron is recommended per day. This should help elevate the body's iron stores postpartum, when it is recommended to get 6.5 mg per day. However, if you are between the ages of 14 and 18, 7 mg of iron per day is recommended. A cup of uncooked spinach has approximately 2.7 mg of iron.

Limitations with breastfeeding can vary based on the baby's sensitivities. However, as a general rule, the breastfeeding mom should limit her mercury intake (tuna, swordfish) and limit her caffeine intake to less than 300 mg (2-3 cups of coffee) per day. Recreational drugs and cigarette smoking should be avoided entirely with breastfeeding so as to not pass dangerous and addictive substances to your baby.

Water intake is very important with breastfeeding as well. It is so important to stay hydrated in order to be able to produce adequate milk. Experts recommend about a gallon daily! That's about 128 ounces per day. That may seem like a lot, but this can be accomplished by keeping a water bottle with you at all times and sipping on it consistently as the day goes on. Another strategy is to drink a cup of water every time you breastfeed. This will help to keep up your supply and keep you hydrated.

> *Breastfeeding water intake is recommended at one gallon per day to produce adequate milk supply (not part of the bookl like the rest, just what I want blurbed to side)*

NUTRITION FOR POSTPARTUM WEIGHT LOSS

I think one of the more important parts of this chapter and the theme of this book is going to be loving your body in a way that honors what it just did. All too often, we see the media glorify celebrities who "bounce back" to whatever crazy body standard is being promoted in the clickbait article they are trying to push.

Those standards are a hot, steaming pile of BS. Why is the media obsessed with women's bodies during and after pregnancy anyway? Get away, creeps.

We really should not be excessively limiting our caloric intake with the goal of significant weight loss for the first three months postpartum. The body needs those calories and nutrients to help itself heal and return to its non-pregnancy state. Lactating mothers really should not be limiting their calories throughout the duration of breastfeeding, either.

It's better to choose healthy foods with higher-quality vitamins and nutrients and make sure you are getting enough of them for your daily energy requirements and for lactation if you are breastfeeding. When I refer to energy requirements, I'm not only referring to if you feel wiped out during the day but also to the energy requirements on a cellular level.

Our bodies are slowly rebuilding. Additionally, with lactation, many will report that their supply drops when they do not eat enough calories throughout the day.

So, calories are crucial.

When that three-month period ends, you're able to ramp up your exercise and physical activity and can start to tweak your nutrition if you still desire weight loss.

It is recommended to try and lose 1-2 pounds per week. This can be achieved by limiting calories gradually—300-500 calories less per day—paired with physical activity for at least 30 minutes five times per week.

The body responds more favorably to this slow, gradual approach, and mentally, it is more likely to become a habit and part of your lifestyle. In other words, your results are much more likely to stick!

When I was postpartum with my second child, I had a nutrition coach for accountability and strategy. When I had my first meeting with him, I told him that my goals were mainly to optimize my eating habits for general improved performance.

Now, when most people hear "improved performance," it may make you think I am some kind of athlete. This is not the case. Last week, I hit myself in the face with a wall ball at CrossFit. No one is sending me to The CrossFit Games.

When I meant performance, I meant "in general" as a human. How could I use nutrition to optimize my energy levels, cellular healing, and overall immunity? What about my mindset and relationship with food?

*How could I use my own nutrition habits to create
examples and model eating good foods for my daughters?*

I wanted them to see a healthy relationship with food and a healthy perspective of body image that has nothing to do with what my body looks like or what number is on the scale—because those last two things don't matter, especially when raising little girls.

When it comes to postpartum weight loss, my best advice is to change your relationship with food in small increments. Week one, add more water intake. Week two, add more vegetables and fruits. Week three, limit your carbohydrates. My nutrition coach and I worked on methods just like these, and he called it "playing offense and defense." Consume more of the good and less of the bad gradually over a good time span to create good habits.

I'm sorry If you got to this section and thought, "Oh good, she's going to tell me what to eat to lose weight." This is definitely NOT that kind of book. Quite frankly, screw bouncing back. I don't bounce anywhere—I arrive with style and attitude when I am ready to get there. Society and the media need to meet us at a place where health and self-love are the sexiest things out there.

CHAPTER SIX:

Parenting Like a Boss

There are so many things that I was unprepared for with becoming a mom. For example, no one tells you how often your kid will try to get into the dishwasher. Enjoy never being able to unload that bad boy without the threat of a small human racing towards the stand-up bathtub inside of the counter to try and stab themselves with the cutlery. They move pretty fast. It's alarming.

I have no authority in this chapter. When I had my first kid, I walked around with imposter syndrome, wondering why the people in charge let me take home a whole baby unsupervised.

There were so many things to figure out while just surviving and figuring out who I was as a new mother.

So, that being said, I don't have any life-changing advice, just funny anecdotes and that same central theme of self-kindness.

The newborn vortex is definitely your initiation period to parenthood, getting hazed by your infant. Lots of crying, very little sleeping, and just when you think the last thread of your mental sanity is going to snap, that little angel nestles their head onto your chest and falls asleep with the tiniest little breaths, and it just resets your soul. It's really hard, but you just keep going, and you make it through it another day, then another—and eventually, you're in the swing of things. You start handling it like a pro, just in time for some brand new parenting crisis to begin and repeat the learning curve process for something new.

Both of my children were sleep terrorists. My oldest would get up many times throughout the night and would often spit up her entire bottle each time. I had to keep three sets of pajamas ready for each of us every night and kept spare bedding nearby in case she duped me and waited until I put her down, pretended to be back asleep, and then blam-o! Formula puke all over her and the sheets. If you don't already know, the horrors of formula puke will haunt you until the end of your days. It is a texture that is not of this world.

A friend gave me the most amazing parenting tip for overnight accidents, getting sick, etc.: buy several crib mattress protectors and sheets, and layer them so that you only have to take off the top protector and sheet. As a safety note, I waited to do this until the kids were a little older in order to abide by safe sleep criteria. However, this came in handy with overnight potty training, too!

My youngest would not get up as many times; however, she would not go right back to sleep and refused to lie down while still awake to fall asleep on her own. This resulted in me being with her no less than an hour and a half each time she got up in the night to rock her all the way back to sleep. I had plenty of time to binge Netflix and eat snacks in this overnight scenario. I was a mom vampire, albeit a mom vampire that was caught up on all the hot Netflix new releases.

I do look back on it as a very special time in my life, one that I wouldn't trade for more rest or free time.

During the infant phase, a lot of advice concerning sleep is out there. Typically, your newborn will take naps throughout the day, which become less frequent as they get older until the toddler stage, where they wean down to about one nap per day. Something that we found very helpful until our oldest was about 4 was the "wake window" schedule. A wake window is a specified amount of time to have your baby awake before laying them down for a nap or bed. We also made sure to get the babies lots of sunlight during the day (even meaning open window shades during nap time) and to keep their rooms nice and dark at nighttime in order to assist with their natural sleep/wake cycles and melatonin regulation. I can assure you that at least one (well-meaning) person is going to let you know that your baby has "their days and nights mixed up" if your kiddo is up all night and sleeping during the day. Sometimes, they just do that.

Another important aspect of safe and restful sleep is a primo swaddle. Up until the baby is able to roll over on their own, it is recommended to swaddle your baby's arms and legs to recreate a secure environment similar to the one they experienced in the womb. A good swaddle can mean more sleep for both baby and mom, which is the name of the game here. Once they are able to roll around, it is no longer safe to secure the arms, and there are a lot of transitional swaddling options. Between both children, we have tried them ALL.

Going out in public with an infant is a circus. A diaper bag for a single outing must contain diapers, wipes, butt cream, bottles, extra formula, snacks, extra clothes for both baby and mom, infant Motrin (just in case), a swaddle, a mini portable baby fan, binkies, stuffies, sound machines, a first aid kit, water, and literally all of your sanity. Don't forget your stroller and car seat cover so strangers can't breathe their adult-sized germs on your miniature human being.

I have often wondered why people feel the need to get super close and touch your baby. Of course, babies are cute and sweet, and we want to "oooh and ahh" over the little sweet peas; however, do it from a distance, please, and thanks.

Do you feel like you are a non-confrontational person and panic at the thought of having one of these interactions? If so, I have compiled a list of things to say to someone getting too close: "Whoa, watch out! She took off the last person's finger in one clean bite!" or "Sure, you can look in and say hi, I don't think he's contagious anymore" are some great options.

All joking aside, you don't owe anyone anything when it comes to your child, not strangers, not family members, not anyone.

The fact of the matter is that you and your partner need to make the decision regarding what is in your comfort zone and when you're comfortable letting your baby be exposed to other people.

We had our first baby pre-pandemic, and even though the pandemic made me a lot more germ conscious, I was still pretty strict with germ exposure to my children before they were eight weeks old and got their first round of vaccinations. Following that time, both kids went to daycare and got ALL of the germs. That being said, they do have pretty good immune systems now.

COMPARING YOUR BABY TO SOMEONE ELSE'S KID
Every baby develops and hits milestones at their own pace. This is another one of those irrational things to worry about when you compare your baby to your nephew, who walked out of the birth canal and was doing calculus before he could eat solid foods.

Milestones exist to help guide us into not missing big red flags with development. The CDC has charts for different time periods to help guide what's typical for growth and development. They are not a perfect timeline, just a sort of safety net criteria to make sure babies are on track. Not walking by 12 months? It's okay. They will get there, and if you have any serious concerns, that's what your pediatrician is there for! Ask them. There are pediatric physical, occupational, and speech therapists who all specialize in this kind of stuff and are happy to help and answer your questions! Reach out! Most likely, though, it all comes down to kids developing on their own timelines.

People love to brag about their kids. It's awesome to be proud of your progeny and let everyone know it, but sometimes parents can glorify or exaggerate with their rose-colored parent glasses on. If your kid didn't crawl or sit up as fast as their baby prodigy did, that's okay—you're doing a great job, and your baby is doing a great job.

> *Don't let that comparison steal your enjoyment of watching*
> *your kid learn how to react to the world around them.*

It's so cool that we get to be a part of that and help to influence that.

RETURNING TO WORK VS. STAYING AT HOME

Maternity leave never feels like enough time. Most women get 8-12 weeks paid time off—maybe—and if dad gets paternity leave, it's practically a miracle. Compared to other countries around the world, the US is pretty paltry with doling out time off for increasing the census with your miniature human. Most women are still physically healing at that time, they definitely aren't sleeping through the night, and they emotionally have just gone through an extremely significant change. Returning to work is tough and presents these, among many more challenges. Moms are superhumans and pull this off without much of a fuss. Having to go back to work, especially at eight weeks postpartum, is heartbreaking because the baby is so small. You've just spent two months existing to attend to this person; how can you leave them now? It's devastating.

According to a list comprised by the Organization for Economic Co-operation and Development (OECD) comparing maternity leave across different countries, Greece comes out on top, guaranteeing full pay for 26.6 weeks of work. They also guarantee 43 weeks of maternity leave and, on average, pay 61.8% of mom's salary. Would you care to wager a guess as to how many weeks the US guarantees for paid maternity leave?

If you guessed zero, you would be depressingly correct.

Yes, we do have the Family and Medical Leave Act (FMLA), which requires employers to give eligible employees up to 12 weeks off, but it does not require them to pay the employee. Companies with under 100 employees are exempt from FMLA altogether. That's bleak. Europe has us beaten by a long shot on this—we aren't even in the race. At any rate, whether you get paid or not, eventually, that day is going to come when, if you are returning to work, it will be time to drop your sweet love bug off at daycare or your other source of childcare, and it will never feel like they are old enough to be out in the world on their own without you!

The first day of daycare drop-off is going to be tough. I cried with both. I have seen other parents standing outside crying together after day one drop-off and felt that deeply. I wanted to include this portion to tell you that you don't have to be strong—that is going to be a REALLY HARD day. Take an extra-long car ride to work, park, and flip through your favorite pictures of your baby and your family. You will get through it.

Some people talk about a divide between mothers who stay at home with their children and those who return to work.

I want to be clear that these two factions of women—those who go back to work and those who stay at home—are BOTH superheroes in their own ways.

Both have to make hard sacrifices to do what they think is best for their family's situation. The working mother aches for her children's hugs and laughter during the work day, but maybe their family cannot survive without the income, or maybe her work fulfills her passion for something wonderful in the world and allows her to grow as a person and leader. The stay-at-home mom often may feel like her life revolves around her little one's every need and that she loses her identity in the process, yet she loves that she has the ability to stay and nurture her child's development.

There are challenges for both moms, and there are wonderful aspects as well. Both moms work very hard to make the world a better place for their kids, which is why I find myself getting a little salty when someone makes a flippant criticism of either.

When I returned to work after the birth of my first child, a woman of an older generation was shocked and asked me, "Well, where is the baby?" I responded kindly that she was at a very lovely daycare, to which the woman responded, "Well, she's never going to know you!" Me being the type of person who defers any social discomfort with self-deprecating humor, I told her that I was not sure, but my little one seemed to recognize me from time to time, and I would work on it with her with some flashcards with my picture on them. It was surprising to me, with both kids, after I returned, how many people were puzzled by the fact that I returned to work and did not stay home. There's also the struggle of scrambling to navigate sick days, missing school parties because of work, and just the general feeling of not having enough time in the day to spend with your kids. It can be overwhelming.

The emotional uphill battle of going back to work would be hard enough to tackle on its own, but working conditions are not always great, especially for breastfeeding mothers who typically need a private space and time to perform pumping out that liquid gold to send with their babies to daycare.

There are two federal laws that protect many women in the workplace—the Break Time for Nursing Mothers and The PUMP Act, which wentill go into effect in April of 2023—which both essentially state that women are to be provided a private space that is not a bathroom and break time (paid or unpaid) to pump.

These will protect the pumping mother for up to one year following the birth of their child.

Even though there are some laws in this country about pumping at work, a lot of women feel like they are not able to take the break required to do so without falling further behind on their work. They are supposed to be given a safe and private place to pump, but some get stuck in a supply closet, sitting on a milk crate and crouched over a laptop, humming away to the lulling sounds of their Spectra. In recent years, I have seen and heard about companies adding great spaces for women to pump in private and also get some work done, but the mental tug-of-war between being an efficient mom vs. an employee can often cause feelings of guilt for the new mom in both directions. What if you're a kindergarten teacher or a nurse with minimal time to squeeze in a bathroom break, let alone a pumping break? The choices we have to make are constant and hard.

Even now that my kids are a little older, the days vary. Some days, I have a hard time, and I really miss them all day long, and some days, I am so grateful for the ability to take a lunch break all by myself and sit in silence for an uninterrupted 30 minutes.

The stay-at-home mom is often undervalued when, in fact, they are a crucial part of the household—the heartbeat of a home. A survey performed states that the average work week of the working mom is 106 hours ("Salary.com").

If we were to pay the working mom for all of her duties on average with what childcare, housekeeping, cooking, etc., would cost, it would come to $184,820.

I wonder if that figure is also subject to the glass ceiling and if stay-at-home dads would be estimated at a higher number. But I digress.

The feedback I have encountered from stay-at-home moms includes loss of identity and never having any time to themselves because they are always "on" in order to take care of their tiny human and family. They are the safety net that has to remember all of the things: pediatrician appointments, put dinner in the oven by 4:30 so it's ready when dad gets home, turn over the laundry while the baby naps, etc., etc. It never ends. The juggling of childcare and homemaking is tough.

Both sets of moms are placed under unrealistic pressures to get everything done and simply do not have enough hours in the day to do all of the things necessary—something often needs to be sacrificed. For example, my house is always a mess, and I have clutter piles all about. If you come to my house, it is known that this place is lived in—which is my euphemism for it being a mess—and I did not have the mental bandwidth to clean up.

No matter if you stay home or go back to work, it was likely a difficult decision that was not made lightly. To me, it's a really great example of the strength demonstrated by moms every day.

WORKING AS A TEAM WITH YOUR PARTNER

Relationships are all unique, and each is vastly different from the next, but a universal truth about having a baby with your partner is that it is going to change things significantly. Roles are going to change, and it is going to put a healthy strain on things. Navigating this change with your partner has the opportunity to bring you closer than ever. There are also a lot of opportunities to feel negative feelings like anger, resentment, isolation, neglect, and frustration.

> *There is a huge new set of responsibilities and duties to share, as well as the mental and physical toll that raising a child will take on both of you.*

I used the word "opportunity" because when it comes to communication with anyone else, you essentially are making a conscious choice about how you act and react to things. Some days, it is easier to choose peace over choosing anarchy, and some days, it may take everything in your power to stop considering pouring a bucket of cold water on your spouse when they sleep through yet another time in the middle of the night when the baby wakes up and needs a bottle.

I have a lot of moms who come in frustrated and feeling resentful toward their partners because they feel isolated, overworked, and misunderstood. A good amount of the time, once they get some things off their chest, they feel a lot better and work out a few things that they can go home and discuss with their partners about their feelings.

I am by no means a qualified couples counselor, but I am a huge fan of couples counseling in hard times, in good times, in sad times, and everything else under the sun. It is strongly supported that couples take time for themselves to work on their relationship and their communication after this big life change.

Put love in and get more love out instead of just secretly hoping your baby has a MASSIVE blowout all over your partner when they are holding them.

There are so many firsts to navigate, some of them good and some of them scary. Mother's intuition is a real thing; listen to it. But also remember that no one has the right answer all of the time and to give yourself grace. Enjoy the highlights and the mundane day to days and know that the hard days will come, but you will keep on trucking through to the other side of it.

There are SO MANY DIFFERENT OPINIONS on how to raise your children. I am going to let you in on a secret: all of the Instagram influencers want you to believe that their method is the best. Perhaps there is a class they want to sell you on this method they believe to be best. Your mother, in-laws, and even cousin Becky all have suggestions on how they did it when their child was a baby, but the big secret is that none of us have the right answer or the magic cure for whatever the issue is. We are all just doing the best we can.

There is already a lot of stress that comes with being a parent, so try not to allow someone else's opinion to make you feel judged.

When you think about the big picture, your baby is not going to be little for long. I am not saying this to inspire panic or to give you a lecture about "savoring being a mother." It's just the bittersweet fact that accompanies watching your child grow up. It happens too fast for all of us. Just be there, love them, and love yourself in the process. When I think about that concept in my parenting, I think about Jim and Pam's wedding day from "The Office," when they decide to pretend to take snapshots of the little moments they don't want to forget. Take that snapshot and tuck it away in your heart to warm it to help cushion the blow of moments when your child takes all of their clothes off at a birthday party despite you pleading with them to keep their pants on while wrangling their little sister.

Just remember: you're doing a great job, you've got this, and your kids are lucky to have you loving them in the way that only you can!

We covered a lot of ground in this book. There are a lot of aspects of life postpartum that were surprising to me and things that I have discussed frequently with other moms, too. This book isn't exhaustive of everything that happens in that time period. The span of physical changes and emotional changes is vast, and the experience is so personal for each individual mom and their child.

I wanted to bring a theme of community, most of all, in the sense that I wanted people to be able to connect to these words and experiences and not feel alone.

I hope this book is able to speak to new mothers, make them feel seen, and give them permission to love themselves for doing their best.

Thank you for joining me on this journey and reading this book. Now, go enjoy your baby and your family—I hope you get lots of love, joy, and laughter along the way.

WORKS CITED

Christopher, Shefali, et al. "Rehabilitation of the Postpartum Runner: A 4-Phase Approach." Journal of Women's Health Physical Therapy, vol. 46, no. 2, Feb. 2022, pp. 73–86. https://doi.org/10.1097/jwh.0000000000000230.

Gammill, Hilary S., and J. M. Nelson. "Naturally Acquired Microchimerism." The International Journal of Developmental Biology, vol. 54, no. 2–3, University of the Basque Country, Jan. 2010, pp. 531–43. https://doi.org/10.1387/ijdb.082767hg.

Rijnink, Emilie C., et al. "Tissue Microchimerism Is Increased During Pregnancy: A Human Autopsy Study." Molecular Human Reproduction, vol. 21, no. 11, Oxford UP, Nov. 2015, pp. 857–64. https://doi.org/10.1093/molehr/gav047.

Salary.com. "Moms: We Know You're Worth It. But How Much Is 'It' Really Worth?" Salary.com, 22 Jan. 2019, www.salary.com/articles/stay-at-home-mom.

"Screening for Perinatal Depression." ACOG, www.acog.org/clinical/clinical-guidance/committee-opinion/articles/2018/11/screening-for-perinatal-depression.

REFERENCES

Avena, Nicole M., PhD. What to Eat When You're Pregnant: A Week-by-Week Guide to Support Your Health and Your Baby's Development. Ten Speed Press, 2015.

"Breastfeeding Support and Resources Toolkit." AAFP, www.aafp.org/family-physician/patient-care/prevention-wellness/birth-control-pregnancy-childbirth/breastfeeding/toolkit.html#:~:text=Breastfeeding%20Support%20and%20Resources%20Toolkit%201%20A%20Healthy,Science%20%26%20Education%20Importance%20of%20Growth%20Charts%20.

"CDC And Breastfeeding." Centers for Disease Control and Prevention, 19 Jan. 2023, www.cdc.gov/breastfeeding.

Chauhan, Gaurav. "Physiology, Postpartum Changes." StatPearls - NCBI Bookshelf, 14 Nov. 2022, www.ncbi.nlm.nih.gov/books/NBK555904.

"Diet Considerations for Breastfeeding Mothers." Centers for Disease Control and Prevention, 17 May 2022, www.cdc.gov/breastfeeding/breastfeeding-special-circumstances/diet-and-micronutrients/maternal-diet.html.

Durnea, Constantin M., et al. "Prevalence, Etiology and Risk Factors of Pelvic Organ Prolapse in Premenopausal Primiparous Women." International Urogynecology Journal, vol. 25, no. 11, Springer Science+Business Media, Apr. 2014, pp. 1463–70. https://doi.org/10.1007/s00192-014-2382-1.

"FLSA Protections to Pump at Work." DOL, www.dol.gov/agencies/whd/pump-at-work.

Goom, Tom, et al. "Returning to Running Postnatal – Guidelines for Medical, Health and Fitness Professionals Managing This…" ResearchGate, Mar. 2019, https://doi.org/10.13140/RG.2.2.35256.90880/2.

Iglesia, Cheryl B. "Pelvic Organ Prolapse." AAFP, 1 Aug. 2017,

www.aafp.org/pubs/afp/issues/2017/0801/p179.html.

Malhotra, Anita, et al. "A Stepwise Approach to Prescribe Dietary Advice for Weight Management in Postpartum and Midlife Women." The Journal of Obstetrics and Gynecology of India, Springer Science+Business Media, Mar. 2022, https://doi.org/10.1007/s13224-022-01643-w.

Martin, Julie P., et al. "Postpartum Diet Quality: A Cross-Sectional Analysis From the Australian Longitudinal Study on Women's Health." Journal of Clinical Medicine, vol. 9, no. 2, MDPI, Feb. 2020, p. 446. https://doi.org/10.3390/jcm9020446.

Nygaard, Ingrid, et al. "Early Postpartum Physical Activity and Pelvic Floor Support and Symptoms 1 Year Postpartum." American Journal of Obstetrics and Gynecology, vol. 224, no. 2, Elsevier BV, Feb. 2021, p. 193.e1-193.e19. https://doi.org/10.1016/j.ajog.2020.08.033.

Prevett, Christina, et al. "Impact of Heavy Resistance Training on Pregnancy and Postpartum Health Outcomes." International Urogynecology Journal, Springer Science+Business Media, Nov. 2022, https://doi.org/10.1007/s00192-022-05393-1.

Selman, Rachel, et al. "Maximizing Recovery in the Postpartum Period: A Timeline for Rehabilitation from Pregnancy through Return to Sport." International Journal of Sports Physical Therapy, 17 Jun. 2022: 1170-1183.

Skaug, Kristina Lindquist, et al. "Prevalence of Pelvic Floor Dysfunction, Bother, and Risk Factors and Knowledge of the Pelvic Floor Muscles in Norwegian Male and Female Powerlifters and Olympic Weightlifters." Journal of Strength and Conditioning Research, vol. 36, no. 10, National Strength and Conditioning Association, Dec. 2020, pp. 2800–07. https://doi.org/10.1519/jsc.0000000000003919.